Good Morning Gorgeous

Keys to Discovering Your "Gorgeousness" From the Inside Out

Dale Smith Thomas

Published by Franklin Green Publishing
P.O. Box 51
Lebanon, Tennessee 37088
www.franklingreenpublishing.com

Printed in the United States of America

ISBN 978-1-936487-40-0

Cover Photo: Kristy Belcher
Cover and Interior Design: Bill Kersey, www.kerseygraphics.com

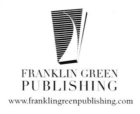

FRANKLIN GREEN
PUBLISHING
www.franklingreenpublishing.com

This book is dedicated to:
To all the gorgeous spirits who are
looking to discover themselves and
find out they are truly gorgeous,
inside and out!

A SPECIAL MESSAGE FROM DALE

First of all, I want to say a heartfelt thank you for picking up this book and entering this Good Morning Gorgeous journey with me. I truly believe that if this book is in your hands, then you and I are on a date with destiny. There is something here for you: from lessons that can guide you to another portion of your life to ideas that can unlock that gorgeous, unique potential that only you possess in order to help you live your dreams.

I can tell you that writing every word of this book and creating each segment has been a labor of love. This is my second book, and to be honest, I imagined that this time around I would just sit down and write this book quickly. It has been several years since my last book was published. Since then, I have had so many amazing life experiences. I have spoken to audiences around the world, met many fascinating individuals, and listened to the personal stories of thousands of people. It has been my honor and pleasure to work with some of my mentors and people whom I previously admired from afar, including Dick Clark, Zig Ziglar, Les Brown, Dr. Phil, and many more. Through the years, I have journaled and documented the lessons I have learned from those experiences and the lessons I have learned through life that I now teach. I truly thought this book was going to be easy to write.

It was not. Far from it.

Writing this book has been one of the hardest things I have ever done. Each time I thought the manuscript was *done,* something would happen that became another lesson that I had to share. Writing certain portions of this book made me come face to face with insecurities that I thought had already been battled and won. I had to learn that this book was not just going to come *from* me; it had to come *through* me to be effective in your life.

The phrase *Good Morning Gorgeous* at first glance could seem superficial and all about the outer appearance, but nothing could be further from the truth. I can honestly say that growing up I never felt "gorgeous." I had hair that I wanted to be straight that just got bigger with the Mississippi humidity. I had big eyes and big lips and was too tall and too skinny all at the wrong time. My teenage years, and even into my twenties, I struggled with low self-esteem and a very negative self-image. There was very little I liked about myself. As you will read later, that negative view of myself led me to the brink of a serious illness. Only the life lessons from great teachers and finally learning to trust myself brought health, healing, and the life I now live as a teacher, speaker, and author.

You will notice that I did not divide this book into chapters. I have divided it into "gifts," because these seven principles are the lessons that have truly been the gifts in my life, and I pray that as you read these ideas and lessons they will also be gifts to you. In addition, make sure you look for the information in Gift Seven on how to receive a special gift I would like to mail to you. You will also notice that we have created many spaces for you to basically use this book as a workbook. I am an avid reader, and I always have a notebook with me when I read to write down my personal takeaways. We have created that space for you at the end of each chapter. I hope you will not only read, but you will also use those spaces to help you internalize these messages.

My sincere desire is that by the time you "work" (and I hope you do work) through this book, you will truly grasp and understand that true beauty, and being uniquely gorgeous, can only come from one place: within. I hope that as you read these words they will not be just information to you but will transform your soul inside and out. I pray that you will start to discover how truly special you are and begin to understand that we all came to this earth with an invisible crown of value and self-worth on our heads. It's a crown than can get lost along the way. This book will help you find that crown again. No one on this planet has your gifts, your talent, and your gorgeous spirit. It's time to be all you were created to be—not only for yourself, but as an encouragement to others.

I invite you to join me in a movement to spread the *Good Morning Gorgeous* message around the world to help others discover their true value. I welcome you to become a Good Morning Gorgeous Disciple, a Good Morning Gorgeous Ambassador, and an active part of our Good Morning Gorgeous Tribe. My heartfelt desire is that as you uncover your gorgeous soul, you will help others do the same. I believe that together we can create a ripple effect that will encourage other women around the world to be all they were created to be!

So regardless of your age, height, weight, race, or gender, I say to you "Good Morning Gorgeous!" I am here with you through the pages of this book as your coach, your mentor, your friend, your soul sister, and your guide to encourage, challenge and inspire you to rise up to your greatest potential. Crowns up my friends, Welcome to the Good Morning Gorgeous Family!

With Love,
Dale

HERE'S TO THE WOMAN
...who knows where she's going
and will keep on until she gets there;
who knows not only what she wants from life
but what she has to offer in return...

HERE'S TO THE WOMAN
who is loyal to family and friends,
who expects no more from others
than she is willing to give;

HERE'S TO THE WOMAN
who guides and inspires
not by quoting others philosophies but by living
her own good example;
who accepts both victories and disappointments
with the same grace,
and who can rise above life's
challenges and move on...

HERE'S TO THE WOMAN
who gives the gifts of her thoughtfulness, who
shows her caring with a word of support,
her understanding with a smile; a woman who
brings joy to others just by being herself...

~ AUTHOR UNKNOWN ~

Good Morning Gorgeous Gifts

Gift One : Discover Your Beauty   11

Gift Two: Change Your Mind   31

Gift Three: Listen To Your Soul   57

Gift Four: Find Yourself – Know Yourself   89

Give Five : Uncover Your Dream   115

Gift Six: Turn On The Light   141

Gift Seven: Chin Up, Crown Up   163

Acknowledgments   186

About the Author   187

66 That's the thing about inner beauty: unlike physical beauty, which grabs the spotlight for itself, inner beauty shines on everyone catching them, holding them in its embrace, making them more beautiful too. 99

GIFT ONE

Discover Your Beauty

#GMG

Pretty Is . . .

Good Morning Gorgeous! Good Afternoon Gorgeous! Good Evening Gorgeous! In the words of two precious little girls, daughters of one of my best friends, Brooke and Braden, "Oh My Gorgeous!" Regardless of what time of day you have decided to join me with this book—the one word, the one theme you are going to hear through this journey, is *Gorgeous*. I don't even remember when I first started teaching and sharing this message; however, it has been a central theme I have shared around the world—a "mantra" and a challenge for many people.

I have honestly been surprised and encouraged at what a difference these three little words can make in someone's energy and attitude. When I share this message from the stage, I ask my audience members to turn to each other and simply say, "Good Morning Gorgeous." Instantly, they begin smiling and laughing, and the entire energy in the room elevates to a new level—it's a simple, positive affirmation that encourages and brings a smile to someone's face.

As I said in the introduction, this is going to be a journey. A journey into inner space. A journey that will have you battling all the old messages that have kept you hidden inside yourself. I want you to think about this: how do you feel if someone says, "Good Morning Gorgeous" to you? I know that for most of my life, it didn't feel real. It didn't fit. I had all the false reasons in my head and heart to back up why that statement wasn't true. I didn't realize at that time that being gorgeous is an attitude and a spirit that must come from the inside and be reflected outside. Maybe you have never felt gorgeous, but I am saying to you right now, you are gorgeous. I do not have to see you to know that you are gorgeous in many ways.

So let's try it. Quick. Put down this book. Find yourself a mirror. Take a look at the person in the mirror and simply say, "GOOD MORNING GORGEOUS!"

How did that feel? Did you instantly feel some resistance from your inner soul? I know from experience that many of your internal voices inside your soul may have already gone into full attack mode with an arsenal of reasons why the word *gorgeous* does not apply to you. Every single person reading this book is gorgeous in her (or his) own way! It is my job to help you find that gorgeous spirit inside of you—release it and learn to celebrate it, regardless of your age, race, size, or gender.

> ❝A gorgeous spirit is about who you are from within, that is simply reflected in your outer appearance. ❞

This book will encourage you, inspire you, and push you to find your personal truth. I will guide you and help you silence that negative voice that resides in all of us. I believe when you uncover, discover, and maybe recover your dynamic spirit that is inside of you, it will challenge you to follow your biggest dreams and help you learn to celebrate your uniqueness. As I share my personal story and stories of others, it is my greatest hope that these stories will remind you that we all face challenges and, at times, criticism along the way. We have all doubted ourselves—our worth, our value, our beauty, our strength, and our ability—at one time or another. We all need someone in our lives to encourage us to be proud of who we are and where life has taken us. If you do not have that person, then *I* am your person through the words of this book.

Each and every situation you and I have faced has a valuable lesson within that experience. Those experiences have the power to alter your life for the best. Embrace your journey, wherever it has taken you. Realize that each life experience brings lessons for you that could only be taught by that experience. For me, it is like my shoe experiences. Anyone who knows me knows that I am a high heel shoe junkie. Each shoe brings me a different experience. I learned quickly in my shoe love that I have some one-hour shoes, some four-hour shoes, some five-hour shoes, very few all-day shoes, and some that just need to sit on the shelf and look pretty.

Why do I do it? Why would I ever wear shoes that I could only stand for one hour? I get asked all the time if my shoes are comfortable; I truly laugh at the question every time it's asked. I need to be clear: I have rarely answered yes to that question. I do it because I love my high heels, and for whatever crazy reason, they make me feel gorgeous. Very few people understand this love connection, but I salute a few of my "sole/soul" sisters who truly do understand—you know who you are!

It's not important to understand my shoe love or to understand my personal journey. It's not important if other people understand your journey either, *but* it is important that you understand your journey. This is about discovering the authentic, real you and being brave enough to never hide from that authenticity again. It's facing the lies that you have been told, both by yourself and others, and once and for all setting the record straight. Your choices may not be right for someone else, but what truly matters is whether those choices are right for you. As my friend Les Brown once said, "Someone else's opinion of you is none of your business." I say, Amen, to that, Les!

66*It's not important if other people understand
your journey. It is important that
YOU understand YOUR journey.*99

So, what does it mean to you to "feel" gorgeous? What immediately comes to mind? Please take a moment and journal in the following spaces what it means to feel gorgeous; just write down the first thoughts that pop into your head. What makes you feel gorgeous? For me, it's my shoes; it's being happy and joyful; it's finding a great dress on sale; it's helping someone else. There are no right or wrong answers. Have fun with this, and remember that feeling gorgeous isn't just about an outward appearance.

Now, what if I asked you "who" do you think is gorgeous—would your name appear on that list? I can tell you from talking to women all around the world that a majority of you said no. It seems that many of us only think the word "gorgeous" applies and is reserved for the top models and actresses in Hollywood; it does not apply to us. One thing I know without a shadow of a doubt is that being gorgeous is not something the mirror reflects; it is truly a state of mind and spirit. I also believe that everyone has gorgeous outer features, but many times we have focused for so long on the things we don't like about our outer appearance that we rarely see the things that are beautiful.

> 66 *Being gorgeous is not something the mirror reflects, but is truly a state of mind and spirit.* 99

I will be honest with you, I did not grow up thinking I was pretty, beautiful, gorgeous, or even cute. Even though I competed much later in life in a "beauty" pageant, I was not one of the childhood beauties who competed in pageants. I grew up on a farm in rural Mississippi. My days were filled bumping down dirt roads in my daddy's old pickup truck going to feed the cows or working in the garden with my momma. I was just a little country girl out on a farm who didn't think she was pretty. I was tall and skinny, had really big eyes, big lips, and a head full of wavy hair. All the things I appreciate now, I did not like growing up. Being a teenager in the 70s, I wanted straight hair, but there was nothing I could do to make that happen. This was long before I knew about a flat iron. I struggled every day not feeling pretty, as I'm sure many of you have.

I was teased about my "big" eyes and "big" lips. Although I don't remember who teased me about those features, I can totally remember what they said, even though it's been over forty years. I am sure you can instantly remember some of the things you were told as a child that were not flattering or kind. Why is it that those are the things we remember? I'm sure I was told some positive things at that time, but those were not the messages I focused on at all.

Research has shown that negative memories are more likely to be remembered than positive memories, because negative events pose a "chance of danger." This makes the body more alert to negative thoughts, because they are treated as a lesson to be learned to prevent you from harm. Negative thoughts get all of our focus, and what we focus on gets bigger. It gets burned into our memory because we give it so much air-time. We obsess about it and build a case against ourselves.

These big, full lips that I was so self-conscious about growing up are now being created in women all over the world with the help of collagen. Yes, I love them now, but as a six-year-old, I didn't think they were very cute. Someone asked me the other day if my lips were real. What they wanted to know was, have I had work done? I laughed and said, "Yes, they are real. They are mine. Shall I show you a picture of my daddy to prove it?"

It took me decades to begin to feel comfortable in my skin. It took walking through some real-life challenges. It took changing my belief system about myself. I began to work on changing my belief system after I graduated from college. I had started to realize how negative I was and that I truly had no idea who I was. So I decided to become a student of life. I began to do the work, and those life lessons that I started working on in my late twenties have dramatically changed my life. They are life principles I still practice every day. The three major principles that began to turn my life around were changing my input, changing the way I talked to myself about myself, and practicing self-discipline.

I will explore these with you throughout this book and help you start to change your internal messages. You are already changing your input, or you wouldn't be reading this book.

One of the first things I started working on was to stop repeating to myself the destructive messages I had embraced growing up. I learned that the words I used to describe myself had power. The words you use to describe yourself have power.

Why do they have so much power? Because your soul is listening. In fact, those words that I repeated to myself and the words you repeat to yourself daily have the most power. Before I started on my personal growth journey, the words I was using were negative. It took time for me to truly grasp that I was the only person who could change that dialogue. I started learning about the effect my "personal view" of myself had on my life. I started telling myself I was "unique" and "distinctive" instead of "skinny as a rail" with "saucer eyes."

At first, saying those words felt weird and foreign, but I stuck with it. I understood it was years of repeating negative messages that had affected me, and I knew I couldn't just change it overnight. It would take the power of repetition. The only way to change an old thought is to implement a new one...a new one that you start to repeat.

If I asked you to tell me the words that you use most to describe yourself, what would you say? I know that we all have automatic go-to words. What are yours? Please take a moment and write in the following spaces a few words that you think most describe you.

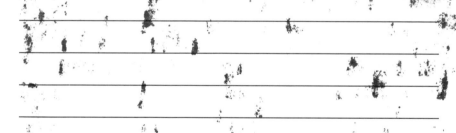

Think about the words you chose automatically. Are they words that make you feel better about yourself or worse? Regardless of the words you chose, I am giving you my two words: unique and distinctive. You are also unique and distinctive, and those are two words you should add to your personal description right now. They may feel unusual to you at first, but they are powerful and strong. The words we use to talk to ourselves on a daily basis have massive, massive power. I am happy to say that most of the words I use to talk to myself now on a daily basis are not discouraging but encouraging, after all these years. But it is still a journey, one that will continue for the rest of my life.

me he doesn't tell me how to speak and therefore I do not have the right to tell him how to do my hair. I just *love* him, and I love my hair! And every woman who is reading this book and has found her perfect "hair relationship partner" knows that no one should try to come between our hair person and us. It will not end well for you!

Now let's talk about "beauty." What *is* it? As I said earlier, if I asked you if you are beautiful or gorgeous, what would you say? Really, what would you say? Is the first word that pops into your mind yes or no? I recently read a study that said that by the age of seventeen, 78 percent of girls in America are unhappy with their bodies. I was shocked and saddened by that statistic. I occasionally get to share my message with teenage girls, and I am blown away at how many of them are already so unhappy with their body image. Recently, one of my friends had a sleepover for her nine-year-old daughter, and she was offering all of the little girls ice cream. She said one of the little girls told her she couldn't eat it because she was on a diet and was on the treadmill every day. What? She's *nine.*

Why is this happening? I'm not an expert in this area, but I believe that even at this young age, these precious little ones are already in the ugly game of comparison with their friends and media images. I have discovered on my journey around the world that this feeling of inferiority and comparison does not have age boundaries. It is common for women of all ages, young and old. An exclusive *Glamour* magazine survey of more than three hundred women of all sizes found that, on average, women have thirteen negative body thoughts daily—nearly one for every waking hour. And a disturbing number of women confess to having thirty-five, fifty, or even one hundred hateful thoughts about their shapes each day. It's not the things that others are saying to us that are harming our self-esteem, it is what we are saying to ourselves.

Think about these statistics, and I mean really think about them

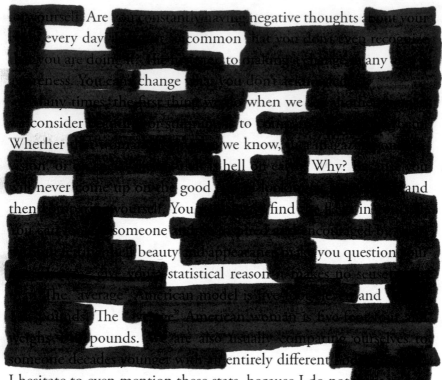

Are ████████████████ negative thoughts about your ██ every day ███████ common ██████████████████ ██ any ███████ You █████ change ███ you don't ████████ █████████████ the first thing █████ when we █████████ ██ consider █████████████████ to ██████████████████ Whether █████████████████ we know, ██████████████ ██████████████████ hell █████ Why? ████████ ███ never ████████████ good ████████████████████ and then █████████████ You ██████████ find ███████ in ███████████ someone ████████████████████████████████████ ████████████████ beauty █████████████ you question ███ ████████████████ statistical reason ████ makes no sense █ ███ average ██ American model is █████████████ and ████████ The ██████ American woman is five feet four █████ weighs ███ pounds. █████████████████ comparing ourselves to ████████ someone decades younger with an entirely different █████████████ I hesitate to even mention these stats, because I do not █████████ compare yourself to them. There isn't a body statistic anywhere that you should compare yourself to—unless it's for your health.

Can you remember a time you compared yourself to someone in a magazine, in a movie, or walking down the street? How did you feel? Did you feel better about yourself or worse? Did it make you celebrate ███████████████████ or did you immediately ██████ to think ████████████████████ wrong with you. I read ██ ███████████ that ██████████████████████████ fashion █████████ for ███ three ████████ ███ 70 ███████████████ ██ 70 ████████ of ████ The girls ████████████████ just ████████ ████████ not to ████████ feel bad ████████████ ████████████████████████ We have to stop ██████

personal assault. The assault isn't coming from the models or the magazines. The assault is coming from within, and anything from within we can change. If we don't like anything about ourselves, we either need to change it or get happy with it. We have to stop this complete self-esteem assault.

May I Have Your Attention Please?

I believe the first step is to *pay attention* to what we are thinking about ourselves. Awareness is always the gateway to change. We have to become aware of the inner chatter that runs as rampant in our minds as the beauty shop gossip. Just like the beauty shop gossip, most of the things we say to ourselves about ourselves are not true. However, our inner self doesn't know that. It simply accepts the truth you give it. If you feed the lies over and over again, then they will become your truth, and you will remain in that 70 percent that feels so awful about themselves. Pain can only feed on pain. Pain can't feed on joy. Pain can't feed on gratitude. We have to be the guardians of our mind.

So many people live with a tormentor in their head that is constantly attacking them. One negative thought won't change how you feel about yourself, just like one drop of water won't make a difference on a rock. But, if you allow those negative thoughts to continue to recycle and repeat in your mind, they will start to change your view. Again, think about the water. Water that continues to drop onto a rock will eventually erode that rock; it's the same for you. Those negative thoughts will eventually erode your self-esteem and self-worth.

I have to say: the men get it. They don't play this nasty game. My husband, and most men I know, would *never* consider comparing themselves to any of those Hollywood "hotties" who are decades younger. We as women, regardless of our age, will look at the Hollywood beauties and want to run for cover. I challenged a guy the other day and accused him of being cocky, and his immediate response was, "No, I'm just convinced." I just loved it and thought it was amazing. Where did we girls lose our way in the self-esteem, self-image department?

I want to guide you away from what the world tries to "sell us" as beauty and push you and shove you to find it for yourself. I remember the day when I finally looked in a mirror and liked who I saw looking back at me. I was over thirty, and I was finally happy with the woman looking back at me. She wasn't perfect, but I was happy with her. Now being in my fifties, I work hard each day to celebrate who I am. Sure, I have the spider veins, some of the laugh lines, and we'll just never know if there is a gray hair under the blonde thanks to Steven. But I have learned to accept and be happy with each stage of the journey of life.

How do we get to and stay in the place in our minds where we are not damaged by the appearance of another woman who we know looks physically better than we do? Trust me, if you look hard enough, you can always find another woman who is taller, thinner, younger, prettier, richer, and the list goes on.

The first step of self-torture is the one I referred to earlier, that age-old demon of comparison. Every time you start looking at other women and comparing yourself in a negative way, you lose. You lose your focus. What you focus on gets bigger, and if you are focusing on all of your faults, they will continue to magnify in your mind. A decision to be happy in your skin is not a decision that you get to make once. It's a daily decision, a daily journey. Each day you get to look at yourself inside and out and DECIDE if you are going to choose to be happy with yourself or not.

Start today to change your mirror image. What you see is totally

Of all the judgements we pass in life, none is more important than the judgment we pass on ourselves.

NATHANIEL BRANDEN

I believe inner beauty is beauty in it's truest form. When we nurture ourselves, it brings an inevitable, positive transformation.

PAUL ABDUL

Take Aways

_____

_____

_____

_____

_____

_____

_____

_____

_____

_____

_____

_____

_____

_____

_____

_____

Take Aways

_____

_____

_____

_____

_____

_____

_____

_____

_____

_____

_____

_____

_____

_____

_____

_____

_____

_____

_____

_____

_____

Your thoughts are the architects of your destiny.

GIFT TWO

Change Your Mind

#GMG

Mind Games

One of my favorite quotes and phrases is this: "Life is won or lost between your ears." Think about that for a moment. Everything in your life is created twice. Between your ears and between your hours. I had to really think about that when I first read it. Look around the room you are in right now; everything there was first someone's "idea" in their mind before it ever was invented. The light in the room, the book you're holding in your hand, or the electronic device you are reading from right now. It was all someone's thought first. It happened between their ears, and then they went to work to make it a reality.

It's a key to success that I share with my audiences worldwide regardless of their profession. It's truly a *mind game*! What do I mean by that? I believe that all of the things in our lives are simply a result of our decisions. Emerson said it best: "The ancestor to every action is a thought." The thoughts that we have lead us to take action. When you decide to change your mind, your thoughts, you will change your actions and your results.

In the next chapter, we will talk about the words that we use to start our day, words that we use that are our inner critic. But where do those words come from? They come from our inner belief system, and we have to start to change what we believe, which will change what we say, which will change what we see, which will change what we do, which will change how we live. Henry Ford had wise words for us all: "Whether you think you can or think you can't you are exactly right." Your subconscious mind is simply your puppet on a string, and it does what your conscious mind tells it to do. If you begin to focus on and give yourself messages that you really don't want, your subconscious will find ways to support that dominant thought. I recently read that your subconscious only knows how to say yes. Our subconscious agrees with all of the instructions and ideas we hold in our focus. If you tell yourself you aren't beautiful or smart, your subconscious says *yes* and gives you all the thoughts to support that idea. If you tell yourself you'll never get the job, find a mate, live your dream, the answer is *yes,* and again the subconscious gives you all the reasons why. But it works both ways. Tell yourself that you can make a change starting today, you can live a life of victory, you can accomplish your dreams, and the answer is also *yes.*

Your subconscious mind is subjective. It does not think or reason independently; it merely obeys the commands it receives from your conscious mind. Just as your conscious mind can be thought of as the gardener, planting seeds, your subconscious mind can be thought of as the garden, or fertile soil, in which the seeds germinate and grow. Your conscious mind commands and your subconscious mind obeys. Your subconscious simply says yes and accepts every thought that you give it. Just like the ground doesn't have the ability to reject seeds, your subconscious doesn't have the ability to reject your positive or negative seeds. It doesn't care what kind of seeds you plant. If you plant positive, powerful seeds, or if you plant the seeds of doubt, it doesn't have an opinion—it just responds. Your subconscious says to your conscious mind, "Your wish is my command."

When you think a thought long enough, it automatically becomes your "default" thought. Remember when you learned to drive a car? It is a very conscious effort initially, but after a few months, the patterns become so embedded in the brain that the whole action of driving becomes subconscious, or automatic. I ask my audiences when I speak how many of them have ever driven to work and don't remember the drive? I can promise you that almost every hand in the room goes up. You don't have to think about the driving process; it has become automatic.

If we hold a negative thought long enough, then that becomes automatic to us. Simply becoming aware of those thoughts begins the process of changing them. As I said, I grew up on a farm in rural Mississippi, and when it rained and my daddy drove the truck out in the field, it made a rut. When the mud dried, that rut was still there, and it was easy just to continue to drive in that rut. The negative thoughts are creating this rut in your mind, and you can find yourself there without even consciously thinking about it.

When we listen to other people as our authority, we adopt their philosophy of life, their attitudes, and their beliefs. If someone tells us we can't do something, and we accept that thought, their opinion of us becomes our reality. I once heard if you "buy" someone's opinion, then you also buy their lifestyle. Before you accept what someone else says about you or your goals and dreams, I want you to stop and ask yourself if they are living the life you want to live. Are they fulfilling their dreams? Are they positive and productive and living a life of integrity? If not, why would you allow their opinion to have so much power? We get so programmed that we don't know what we want or what we really believe.

When my son Nick was small, I started teaching him about choices and truly believing in himself. I wanted to teach him from an early age to believe in himself and not allow anyone's opinion of him change his view of himself. I will never forget the day that Nick and I had gone to a college campus to pick up our babysitter. She was running late, so Nick was standing up on my console through the sunroof yelling hello to everyone who walked by. He was this adorable little chubby-faced boy yelling, "Hi, my name is Nick." Each of the students who walked by would smile, wave, and say, "Hi, Nick."

Suddenly, I heard Nick yelling a little louder, so I sat up and looked to see this girl walking down the sidewalk and ignoring him. She didn't have headphones on or anything. She simply kept walking, and he kept trying to get her attention. As he started to lean down into the car, I was prepared for him to ask me why she wouldn't say hello to him. I was trying to come up with a response. But I was totally wrong. Nick plopped down into the car, looked at me, and said, "She must speak a different language." He didn't take her ignoring him personally—it had nothing to do with him, he assumed she just didn't understand. I could have cried, it made me so happy that he didn't take responsibility for her actions. He let her actions be her actions. And he was *four*!

Many times, we get lost trying to figure out "what we did wrong" when someone doesn't respond or react the way we think they should respond. We need to take a page from the Nick Thomas four-year-old playbook and let their actions be their actions. We don't have to take anyone's word for it as our truth.

I hope that as you read this book, you don't take my word for it but that you let it sink into your soul and you listen to your inner voice and guide to see if these lessons are a fit for you and your life. You have to find your path and the magic in your life. You do that by being true to yourself and listening to yourself. Follow your instinct, your inner guide!

> *You have to find your path &*
> *the magic in your life.*

Over and over again, we read or hear stories of people who have achieved incredible things because they believed. They believed it was possible, and the first step to taking control of your mind is to take control of your belief system.

What do you believe? What do you believe about yourself? Do you believe that you have what it takes to be successful in life? If not, why not? Do you believe that you deserve to be happy and successful, and would you know it if you found it? Do you believe your dreams can come true? If you don't like the results in your life, can you change them? Do you believe you must take 100 percent responsibility for your life? Take a moment and journal what you really believe!

_____

_____

_____

_____

_____

_____

_____

_____

Most people never stand still or get quiet long enough to check in with themselves. They just follow the crowd and follow the direction of someone else. No one thinks in your head but you, and no one can change what you think but you.

You have been overloaded with negative messages your entire life. We grow up being told what we can and can't do, and we carry that into adulthood. We allow the limiting thinking to continue to guide us, direct us, and overwhelm us.

I understand that principle, because I was that person until my mid-twenties. I had to overload the "default" program in my mind, which was negative. I had to stop saying, "I can't" and learn to start saying, "I'll try." I then had to move from "I'll try" to "I will." In other words, I had to change the programming in my brain.

If you truly want to change your internal messages, you have to let go of the thoughts and feelings that are not serving you. You have to reach for "higher ground," a higher feeling, a higher thought. If you want joy, then you have to deliberately release thoughts of sadness. If you want faith, then you must release doubt. If you want victory, then you must release thoughts of failure. Be a detective in your life. What thoughts are your energy vampires? What thoughts always drain you and defeat you? Focusing on the pain of the past is the biggest obstacle for creating a more powerful future. It's very hard for faith to flow through a sea of doubt. It's hard to feel victorious when you are holding onto what you have considered failures in your life. Visualize those feelings that have not served you, and see yourself holding them in your hands in a tight fist. You are holding on so tight. If you want to replace those feelings, those thoughts, and therefore those results with something new, then you have to open your hand and let them go. Release your grip on anything that does not serve you.

Doubt, resentment, anger, frustration, and regret do not serve you. If these thoughts and feelings have gripped your life for a long time, this will not be a one-time process. You may have to say to yourself every day, "I let go of these feelings and thoughts that do not serve me." Once you begin to let them go, you can replace them. You have to add some new information to your mind to overcome all of the negative tapes, messages, and dialogue you have been running for years and years. You have to reject all of the excuses you have made for not living your dreams or even identifying your dreams.

We think in pictures and not in words, and you need to get a visual image of all of the garbage in your mind that leads to "stinkin' thinkin'," as my fellow Mississippian, the late Zig Ziglar, stated. All of those nasty, rotten, obnoxious, dream-robbing messages that live in your mind need to be tossed once and for all. You have to view them as the "garbage" they are and how it directs you every single day. Think about trash for just a minute. What if you never took out the trash? It would be horrible, and it would be toxic.

Think back over the last few days. Have you been buying into the garbage in your mind? Has the dark side been directing your thoughts? I say the dark side, meaning the negative, *nonproductive* side. Darkness will begin to disappear if you flood it with light. However, you have to keep the light on for the darkness to stay away. It won't just go away on its own. You have to turn the light on!

How do you get the darkness in a dark room to disappear? You turn on the light. Get honest. I mean get *really* honest. Do these phrases and words sound familiar? "I'm too old." "I'm too fat." "I'm not smart enough." "I don't have enough money." "No one likes me." "I hate the way I look." "I'm so ugly." "I hate my life." "Why does this always happen to me?" "What is wrong with me?" These words are like a thief in the dark that will sneak up on you and take your spirit and your soul. They will defeat you, and they will keep you paralyzed. Write down the messages you have told yourself that have robbed you and caused you to not follow your heart and dreams. Write down the messages that always make you feel defeated. You have to shed light on the messages that have held you back and release them.

_____

_____

_____

_____

Again, what you focus on gets bigger. I am repeating that phrase over and over to you hoping it will be stuck in your soul. If you understand the true meaning of that one phrase, you *can* change your life! Your mind is a magnet, and whatever you are focusing on you are attracting to you. Do you like what you are getting? If not, **change it!** This is your choice. Release what anyone has said to you in the past that has caused you pain. You do not have to let it be your reality. If someone said something ugly, mean, and hateful to you then, that's their problem. It becomes your problem when you accept it as your reality and start living your life according to their words. It becomes your problem when you hit the "replay" button in your head and repeat that conversation over and over again.

How many times do you repeat the good conversations? Not many, I would bet. It's easier to think about the ugly, nasty, and hurtful things. It keeps us stuck and keeps us playing the blame game, and we don't have to take responsibility for ourselves. I want you to remember that words have power. The words that you speak to yourself and the words that you speak to others have so much power. They have the power to encourage and motivate or devastate and destroy. I remember a story my mother told me about her third-grade teacher that hurts me even to repeat. My mother, who is one of the smartest, most creative women I have ever known, was told by this teacher that she didn't have a thimbleful of sense. That was so cruel. My mother is now in her late seventies and still remembers that was said to her.

People are going to say things to you that hurt you; that is just life. However, stop lying down and rolling over. You don't have to argue with them or get in their face; simply walk away and leave that trash talk in the garbage can where it belongs. That person continues to have power over you *only* if you continue to replay that conversation in your head and base your actions on his or her opinion. So what do you want? Do you want "victory" in your life? Then talk like and think like a "victor"! Do you want success in your life? Then start thinking successfully. I love this quote: "Victims talk about their mountains, but victors talk to them."

If you truly want to change the direction of your life, doing the "soul" work has to be an important part of your daily routine, and it takes as much commitment as the other parts of your life. Think about the things you do every day. You shower, brush your teeth, get dressed, have food, and all of those things are part of your daily routine. Most of them have become automatic. But how much time are you giving your *soul*? It's the self-discipline that I mentioned that changed my life. Personal growth is a daily discipline, and you have to make *improving yourself* a lifelong campaign. I can tell you it's a simple idea that is not easy to practice. It's hard work making the decision to work on yourself every day. I congratulate you; reading this book is part of your soul work. How much fuel are you giving your soul on a daily basis? If you simply gave up ten minutes a day of television, or time on the phone, or time off of social media you could truly start to make a drastic change in your mind, your soul, and therefore the direction of your life.

As busy as I am, I start each day reading something that fuels my soul. I have books everywhere in my house, and I keep different-colored highlighters with me. If I have read a book that spoke to me, I will reread it with a different colored highlighter, because I know it will speak to me in a different way. As we grow and change, the messages speak to us in a different way. Just like we can all feel the effect on our bodies when we don't get enough sleep or have the right kind of food, I can feel the effect on my soul when I have not taken enough time to show up and focus on material that will empower me. I dedicate at least thirty minutes a day to reading and restoring my soul. I urge you to start adding that habit to your daily routine. Are you willing to just redirect thirty minutes each day to your personal self-improvement? Are you willing to feed your soul just thirty minutes each day? Even with a super busy lifestyle, there are so many ways to add powerful messages to your day. There are encouraging messages on YouTube, Instagram, podcasts, and every outlet. Find the one that works best for you, and dedicate that thirty minutes each day. I have two or three go-to books that I know that I can open and find a message of encouragement. I suggest that you do the same.

My team and I read books together and discuss the ideas. We have formed our own book club. If you want to read with us, go to my website, www.DaleSmithThomas.com, and click on the Blog tab and see what we are reading. We would love to know what books are empowering you.

This is your life. This is not a dress rehearsal. Visualize where you want to go, what you want to do, what you want to look like, what you want to give, and what you want to be remembered for. Every time the thief of doubt and destruction tries to play its mind games, you have to hit the STOP button in your mind and play the *victory* tape. Do you have a victory tape? If you don't, you do not have an excuse any longer. You are reading these words, and you have been given the information; now you must act. If you don't act on the information you have been given, then you are no different from the people who did not read this book.

I encourage you to *stop,* my gorgeous friend. I want you to stop, close your eyes, and visualize where you want to go, what you want to do, and what you want to be remembered for. I also want you to stop and begin to think about your Victory List. Your Victory List is the list of things in your life that you are proud of and things you accomplished. It can also be things you are grateful for that have happened in your life—anything that makes you feel stronger, more positive, and more empowered.

Please take a moment and journal in the following spaces what you are grateful for and proud of, right now, today. There are no right or wrong answers. Think about what you have, who you are, and things you have achieved in the past.

This is your **VICTORY LIST**. I encourage you to also record this list on your phone and make it your victory tape!

_____

_____

_____

_____

_____

_____

_____

_____

_____

_____

_____

What is a victory tape? For me, it's several different things. It's the big and small victories in my life; it's the music that empowers me and the friends that I know empower me. You should know the victories in your life. You should write them down and, as I said, record them in your voice. I have a victory playlist made up of songs and lyrics that I know always motivate me. I know the victory friends I can call when I am feeling challenged who will not just listen to me but will lovingly point me back in the direction I need to go.

We are all going to have challenging days, and there are days when we are going to struggle to believe in ourselves. It's called life. However, it's not how many times we get knocked down that matters; it's how long we stay down. Create your victory playlist. Have your victory list of the things you have achieved in your life, and remind yourself of those victories on the tough days. When life knocks you down, remind yourself where you have been and how far you have come. List the times you were brave. List the times that you overcame an obstacle. Go back as far as you need to go. List the times you took action to improve your life. I went all the way back to high school and college when I made my list, because honestly, I didn't see myself as successful during that time in my life. But when I really looked at it today, years later with "new eyes," I could see I was much braver and achieved much more than I gave myself credit for at the time.

Here is the truth: you will see it when you believe it. Read that again. *You will see it when you believe it.* It is the direct opposite of the phrase we have heard over and over again, "I'll believe it when I see it." How do you form a belief? You form a belief by repeating it, focusing on it, visualizing it, and taking action on it daily.

As I mentioned earlier, when I have the opportunity to present at a women's workshop, I ask women to stand up and give me their three best inner qualities and their three outer qualities. I can tell you that 90 percent of the room gets uncomfortable when they are asked to focus on their outer qualities. They can tell you they are a good friend or trustworthy, but ask them to share out loud an outer quality they like, and they wilt. They begin to look around the room for someone to help them with this, and many times I have to point out they have beautiful eyes or hair or a great smile. It really is hard for them to focus on what they like about themselves, and it's harder for them to voice it. However, when I ask them to write down what they want to change, they can instantly write those down. Why? Because every day they reinforce the belief of what they don't like about themselves.

Your inner dialogue can affect everything in your life. Have you ever seen a woman that you thought had a "perfect" body? She had it all, and then you listened to her talk, and all you heard was the things she didn't like about her body. It's all in the mind. Everyone in the world can tell you that you are great, you are beautiful, you have a great body, or you have a great talent, but until you believe it in your mind, it will be idle words and it will fall on deaf ears.

I again think about growing up on a farm. My daddy could not plant a crop if the soil was hard. If he tried to plant seeds in the hardened soil, the seeds would lie on top of the ground and never take root. The birds and animals would come and take those seeds. He had to till the land and get it ready for planting. It's the same in your mind. If the soil in your mind has turned into hardened soil where nothing positive can grow, then you have to till the soil. You have to do the work. Change the type of messages you are feeding your mind and soul. Your mind is not going to change if you keep feeding it all the non-victorious, negative things you have been feeding it. Your image of yourself will not change if you keep saying the same things to yourself every single day. Nothing in your life will change unless you choose new thoughts, new actions, new conversations, and new habits. The good news and bad news is that this is *your* battle and *no one* else's. You can change your input at any moment you choose!

Are you listening or hearing those around you as they speak to you? What do they tell you they like about you? Do you discount it? Do you qualify it? Do you just totally reject it? Please write down what you are hearing and what is being said about you. Once you have completed that, write **DISCOUNT, QUALIFY, REJECT,** or **ACCEPT** after each statement.

_____

_____

_____

_____

_____

_____

_____

I ask this question to many women around the world, and the answer is always the same. I ask, "What do most women do when they receive a compliment?" They usually tell me that it's given back or rejected. We reject the gift of the compliment. I think we do not honor ourselves or the person who has given us the compliment when we reject it and give it back. Many times, when we receive a compliment, we begin to explain why it is not true. How many times have you told someone they looked pretty or nice, and they began to tell you why it wasn't true? We need to simply learn to say thank you and accept that compliment. I really want you to think about it. Ask yourself how you react when someone gives you a compliment. Do you feel strange and uncomfortable? Do you feel like you have to discredit what someone just said to you? Stop sending back the gifts that are being sent to you. When someone gives you a compliment, it is a gift to your soul. Accept the gift. This is a girl thing. I have *never* heard a man discount a compliment. I am sure it has happened, but in my life, if I compliment a man, he thanks me and stands up a little straighter, giving me a little nod that says, "I already knew that."

How many times have you ever complimented a friend only to have her immediately push back and tell you why the compliment isn't true? Her head goes down, her shoulders slump, and her energy pulls inward, and she seems embarrassed or ashamed. Why? It's because she doesn't believe it. Even if you don't believe what has been said to you, it is time for you to stop disrespecting those who are trying to encourage you and start accepting some positive fuel into your soul. Think of this as a gift—if you were giving someone a gift, you wouldn't want them just to hand it back to you. Right now, think about a friend in your life who struggles with this issue. Maybe you struggle with this, and maybe you don't, but I am 100 percent sure that you know someone who does. Call her right now and tell her that you are going to be her "encouraging" mirror until she can see herself for the wonderful, beautiful creature that God created her to be.

If it is you, then I am saying it to you, and I want you to listen to me. "You are a beautiful, wonderful, special creature of God, and you honor and respect no one by being small and talking down about yourself. You are beautiful inside and out regardless of your shape or size." Now say, "Thank you, Dale. I accept these words of encouragement, and I will begin to see myself as God created me and as others see me. I will accept words of victory into my soul."

One of the ways I began to change my life years ago was with affirmations. Honestly, I had no idea what an affirmation was until I read about it. It's simply the statements that you are saying and believing about yourself and your life. It is an agreement, an agreement that you make with yourself. Stating what you want is an affirmation, and a complaint is an affirmation. It's basically an internal form of GPS. You are setting your "aim" through your intention and your words.

Affirmations can be the fuel for your soul and the gasoline for your dreams. It's the energy that will keep you moving forward. Honestly, anything you say, positive or negative, is an affirmation. It's a statement of what you believe. Have you ever heard yourself talking about how exhausted you are, and the more you talk about being exhausted, the more exhausted you feel? That is an affirmation! I have changed my statement from "I'm exhausted" to "I'm in demand." For me, when I talk about being exhausted I feel powerless, but when I say I'm in demand, I feel like I am in control of my choices, which I am. If I am exhausted, it's because I have overloaded my schedule. It's because of the choices I have made. When I talk about being stressed, I feel more stressed. Years ago, I realized what I was doing, and I have changed it to "blessed out," not stressed out. We will always have something in our lives that can stress us out. It is a word that everyone uses. Recently I was so honored to speak for a special event at my parents' little church in Mississippi. I shared this message of changing our language and choosing to be "blessed out." A few days after that event, a mother of a fourth grader posted on my Facebook page a story about her daughter, Mallie, who had been in the service. Her daughter came home from school and told her she had shared what "that lady" had taught at church at school. A little boy in her class had told Mallie that he was stressed out, and she began to share with him that he needed to be *blessed out* instead. She explained to him that we can always choose joy. That story honestly brought tears to my eyes. Being stressed out seems to have no age barriers. Thank you Mallie for being a messenger of hope to others. Each day, I can always find at least one blessing in my life to focus on and so can you. If I am having a challenging day, I choose to believe that it's a *character-building* day instead. Regardless of what we face, we get to choose how we "frame" it.

❝*Affirmations can be the fuel for your soul.*❞

Please take a moment to journal.

List your three "stressed out" phrases that you use. These are your "stressed out" affirmations. They may sound like this: "I'm exhausted," "I'm overwhelmed," "I'm beat," or "I'm so stressed out."

_____

_____

_____

_____

_____

_____

_____

_____

_____

_____

Now list your three "blessed out" affirmations (changing *STRESSED OUT* to *BLESSED OUT*). "I woke up aboveground today, and it's a new day." "I can choose to be happy regardless of my circumstances." "My day is up to me."

_____

_____

_____

_____

_____

_____

_____

_____

_____

I remember when I first heard about affirmations and how weird it felt for me. It's a positive, powerful, present tense, personal, specific statement that should be written down and repeated often. You are placing your order for your life. Your affirmation is not "I will be more positive." Your affirmation is "I am a positive, productive person who is growing and changing daily." It must be in the present tense. When you write down an affirmation and begin with "I will be," that phrase represents something that could possibly happen in the future. When you write, "I am," it gives you power in the present moment. "I am making positive, healthy, choices." "I choose to be joyful today."

One of the stories on affirmations that I love the most comes from the actor Jim Carrey. When Jim was a struggling actor and comic in Hollywood and not making any money, and the offers weren't coming in, he would practice affirmations. He would drive up and sit in his car on Mulholland Drive, look out at the city, stretch out his arms, and say, "Everyone wants to work with me. I'm a really good actor. I have all kinds of great movie offers."

Around 1990, he drove his old Toyota up to Mulholland Drive one night. While sitting there looking at the city below and dreaming of his future, he wrote himself a check for 10 million dollars, dated it Thanksgiving 1995, added the notation, "for acting services rendered," and carried it in his wallet from that day forth. He has stated that it deteriorated, but he saw it in his wallet every day. That visual affirmation helped him build his belief in himself and in his talent. It is no surprise that in November 1995, he found out he was going to earn 10 million dollars for *Dumb and Dumber*. Jim had taken the mental steps and was ready for the manifestation of his dream.

Jim stated to Oprah that he lived in the self-help section at the library. I love that. Jim began changing his internal messages by the information that he was pouring into his soul. Of course, visualization and affirmations must be followed by action. Do yourself a favor and go to YouTube and watch Oprah and Jim's interview from February 17, 1997.

Long before I had read this story about Jim Carrey, I practiced this same philosophy in achieving my goal of winning the Mrs. Tennessee America title. It was my third year to compete, and I had lost both prior years. I went into that third year with a different mindset. I visually closed my eyes every night and saw myself at that competition, and I saw myself walking on that stage, and I saw myself with the crown being placed on my head. I wanted to use the title of Mrs. Tennessee as a platform to start sharing the message of hope and encouragement I had learned through my life. I was thirty years old with a three-and-a-half-year-old son, and I was competing with much younger contestants. It would have been really easy to compare myself to them and talk myself out of the possibility of achieving this dream.

However, because of everything I had learned by becoming a student of life, I practiced my faith, I practiced my affirmations, I worked hard on every phase of the competition, and I truly believed I would be Mrs. Tennessee. When I walked into that competition with more than forty other women, I asked myself how Mrs. Tennessee would act. Would she be nervous, or would she just try to make a difference? If I had already "won," I wouldn't have been nervous, and my goal would be to make a difference.

My roommate at the pageant, Cindy, had never made the top ten when she had competed in previous years. As we talked about the pageant, I asked her what she wanted to achieve, and she told me she just wanted to make the top ten. At that moment, I made it my goal to help her reach her goal. I put quotes and affirmations on the mirror in our hotel bathroom. I sat and helped her write her answer for the top five question. She was sure she wouldn't be in the top five, but I just kept pushing her, and each time she would make a negative comment about herself, I would stop her. We bonded, we laughed, we cried, and in the end, she not only made the top ten and the top five, but she was my first runner up when I was crowned Mrs. Tennessee. As we stood there holding hands and crying, waiting for the winner to be called, we both knew we had already won something much bigger than a sparkly hat. We had helped each other pursue our dreams. She is still one of my dear friends after all these years.

I know it was the "soul work" and the "mind space" that helped make my goal of becoming Mrs. Tennessee America a reality. I know if I had not done the work from the inside out, I would never have achieved that goal. I would have defeated myself before I ever arrived.

Where do you need to change your mind? I lovingly encourage to start to change your mind and start writing down your affirmations. If you cannot write your own yet, then I encourage you to adopt these until you can.

- *I look radiant by simply wearing a smile.*
- *I am a strong woman/man.*
- *I choose to radiate love, joy, and gratitude daily.*
- *I am beautiful, unique, and special.*
- *I have been given a dream; I have the ability to make that dream a reality.*
- *I choose to take action daily to build my inner strength and follow my biggest dreams.*
- *I am gorgeous from the inside out.*
- *I am the champion of my life.*
- *I have the power to change my life.*
- *I am brave, and I am taking steps daily to change my life.*

_____

_____

_____

_____

_____

_____

_____

_____

_____

I AM are two of the most powerful words, for what you put after them shapes your reality.

Anonymous

Everybody is unique. Compare not yourself with anybody else lest you spoil God's curriculum.

Rabbi Israel ben Elieze

Take Aways

_____

_____

_____

_____

_____

_____

_____

_____

_____

_____

_____

_____

_____

_____

_____

_____

_____

_____

" Do not speak badly of yourself. For the Warrior within hears your words and is lessened by them. "

DAVID GEMMELL

GIFT THREE

Listen to Your Soul

#GMG

Stop the Chatter

I love listening to little girls talk, because they are not just talking—they are chattering and giggling. They are like fountains overflowing with joy. On the other hand, when my only child, Nick, was little, he was making truck sounds, gun sounds, and just sounds in general. He never sat and had conversations with his toys. It was all about action and sound. My friends who had daughters tell me they were having conversations with their dolls with full animation. Girls are talking about everything, and I mean, *everything*! It seems that desire to share and "talk about" our lives never changes, even as we mature from our little girl self into a full-blown woman.

Dr. Luan Brizendine of the University of California, who published her findings in *The Female Brain*, says the average woman works her way through twenty thousand words per day, compared with just seven thousand for the average man. A constant state of chatter.

Not a man on planet earth is surprised by this statistic at all. I'm sure they think twenty thousand words a day is an understatement. Every man uses his phone to share the facts, and most women use their phones to share and process. I am sure cell phone companies stay in business because of women. We talk about everything, and now we text about everything. We want to discuss, process, share, and get advice.

Stop Pressing Repeat

Have you ever noticed how women love to repeat, repeat, repeat stories and events? It must be ingrained in our brains from reading it over and over on our shampoo bottles: rinse and repeat. It seems we especially like to repeat stories and situations that tick us off or hurt our feelings, especially if this story involves a man. We need each and every girlfriend in our circle to hear "what he said." I am not sure if it is for clarification or validation. But it seems that we choose to repeat the negative stories much more than we repeat the positive stories. When something happens in our lives and includes drama, it gets a lot of airtime. But it seems we are much more reluctant to share the good news that is happening to us.

Each time you repeat a story or an issue that has caused you any distress, you give it more power and allow it to cause you pain all over again. It is adding fuel to the negative fire that is burning. You get emotionally vested over and over again each time you tell the story. It gains more and more power.

Think about a story that you shared recently more than once with your friends. Was it a positive story or a story about something that had upset you? If it concerned a situation that hurt you, I am almost certain the situation actually happened in a few minutes, but when you repeated it to five friends and felt that emotional pain over and over again—it's as if it happened five more times and a few minutes now have turned into potentially hours of hurt. You are *choosing* to make your life miserable. That is exactly what I just said: *you choose* to make *your life* miserable by hitting the repeat button on those painful experiences.

Have you ever wondered why men get over things so easily and forget them? I can tell you. They don't talk about them. The event happens, whatever the event may be; it concludes; and they consider it done and move on with their day and life.

Trust me, ladies, I think you will find this to be true. When you have a disagreement with your boyfriend, partner, or husband, he is not dialing five of his male friends on the way to work to tell them what you said that hurt his feelings. He will probably tell *no one*! Therefore, by the end of the day, he has forgotten all about it. End of story.

Think about this. You and your partner have a disagreement. He leaves the house and heads for work, and you are still thinking about what he did or didn't say. So you do what we have all done since we were old enough to talk on the phone—you call for backup. After you repeat the story to your girlfriend, she points out some things you hadn't even thought about, and you get even more upset. And what does your partner do? He goes to work and never gives it another thought. He shares it with no one. So when he comes home after a long day at work, he has forgotten all about your discussion, and you are ready to kill him—and he has *no idea* why! Then you are ticked because he forgot! Sound familiar?

This type of cycle is a cycle of self-defeat. It is indeed a self-in-flicted pain. So how do you stop it? It is very simple. Stop adding fuel to a fire that is already burning. Put it out! A fire will not burn without fuel, and you fuel your self-defeating story with repetition. If you need advice and help to find a solution, great—get it. But if you don't want to stay on the pain train, get off! Stop talking and start doing. Logic will never change a wound, but action will. You can't "feel" your way into an action, but you can "act" your way into a feeling. What does that mean? Stop and ask yourself some tough questions instead of just replaying the event in your mind. What can I do *right now* that will change my thought process? What action can I take that will help me feel better?

> 66 *You can't 'feel' your way into an action,*
> *but you can 'act' your way into a feeling.* 99

It has been said that 95 percent of our emotions are determined by the words we choose and the conversations we are having with ourselves. Think about that—really think about that. You are creating the emotional warfare that is causing you distress by the way you "talk" about it.

Remember that your mind can't tell the difference between a real experience and one that is vividly imagined. If you retell a painful story over and over, it is as if it is happening over and over. I have even read that recalling one episode of anger with all of the emotion can depress your immune system for up to seven hours. It is time to stop the insanity!

Here's a rule that I have continued to work on in my life. Spend five minutes identifying the problem in your life, and spend the remainder of the time focused on finding a solution. Spend less time trying to figure out *why* something happened to you and more time on *what* the next steps are to create a solution. Is this easy? No! It's work, and it's hard work, but it's worth it!

Please take a moment and journal in the following spaces the answers to the questions on the next few pages.

What situations and events in your life have really gotten your attention the past month?

_____

_____

_____

_____

_____

_____

_____

_____

What problem(s) in your life have you spent the most time talking about and thinking about this week?

_____

_____

_____

_____

_____

_____

_____

_____

Have you been more focused on the problem or the solution? Define the problem and then give yourself a solution to that problem.

_____

_____

_____

_____

_____

_____

_____

_____

How can you reframe the situation to focus on a better result? What steps can you take to move toward a better result?

_____

_____

_____

_____

_____

_____

_____

_____

Even though I am not an athlete, I am a woman who loves football. I am sure you have all heard the pro athletes "talking trash" to each other. It has always fascinated me to listen to these guys that are wired for sound during a game. They are giving each other all kinds of grief. However, it seems to fire them up and get them ready to go out onto the field and give their best.

Men are weird like that. They can call each other and say the meanest things. But then they laugh at it. The words never mean anything to them personally. I have heard guys joke with each other about their weight, about losing their hair, and about not having dates. They are just talking trash. As women, we would never speak to each other again if we talked trash to each other like men do. Why is that?

I think I have the answer. We don't have to have someone else to talk trash to us, because we are doing it to ourselves. All of the negative messages of doubt are already rampant in our minds, and we don't need anyone else to tell us what they are. I have seen close friends with amazing bodies take a downward spiral just because someone jokingly said, "Have you gained weight?" Words from other people just confirm what we are saying to ourselves. We don't make a habit of talking trash to each other, because we are speaking that garbage into our souls daily.

Women can get up in the morning and, according to the dialogue we choose to speak to ourselves, begin our day in the gutter. It's that nasty little internal voice I mentioned earlier that can defeat us and deplete us before we ever walk out of the bathroom. It's that voice that asks why your hair is so thin, so thick, so gray, so limp, etc. It's that voice when you see the number on the bathroom scale that says, "You will never lose the weight, so why even try?"

The most important conversations you will ever have are the conversations you have with yourself. I challenge you to start to listen to the dialogue that you are constantly giving to yourself. One of the ideas that helped me so many years ago was that I try to *never* say anything to myself that I wouldn't say to a close friend or to my child. Think about this: if you wanted to help your friend, you wouldn't criticize her; you would help her make a positive change. You would direct her to a solution—hopefully, a positive one. If you are encouraging your children, you direct them to see the best in themselves. *We must be the same kind of friend and parent to ourselves.*

I am sure you have read in books or heard on CDs or podcasts about the importance of "self-talk." Book after book has been written about the power of your personal self-talk. Why is it so powerful? Your self-talk acts like your GPS for your life and becomes a self-fulfilling prophecy. You think about it, you focus on it, and your body starts to move in that direction. You set the course in your mind with your self-talk. Again, I think women use their words as assaults to their souls while men use their words to elevate themselves, whether it is valid or not. Recently, while speaking at a conference, the speaker before me stated that women have to be 90 percent sure of themselves before they apply for a job and men only have to be 50 percent sure of themselves.

It's why I started the *Good Morning Gorgeous* campaign. I say it's a campaign because I hope that everyone who reads this not only applies this practice but shares it and becomes part of the **GMG tribe**, the **GMG movement**, and the **GMG family**.

As I travel around the world speaking, I always ask my audiences how they started their day. I am a firm believer that the way we begin our day truly sets the energy for our day. I can ask a room full of people how many of them woke up this morning and looked in the mirror and said, "Good Morning, Gorgeous." Without exception, any time I ask that question, there is always a man in the room who will raise his hand. It makes me laugh out loud, and trust me, everyone in the room laughs. But what I have realized in this very unscientific study is that it's the men who really think that. Men don't usually question if they really look good or not; they just assume that they do. My friend Joe, who is a speaker and author, said an older man he worked with would say this every time he saw his reflection in a mirror, "You are gorgeous, don't you ever change." I laughed so much when I heard this, but I honestly loved it. This man saw his reflection in a mirror and chose only to believe one opinion: his!

Most of the women I have spoken to have told me they get up and look in the mirror and say, "Oh, good gosh." They start the day noticing the things they feel are wrong about their appearance. They are immediately drawn to everything they don't like about themselves. Those imperfections, and the things they don't like, get their full attention.

> 66 *The way we begin our day truly sets the energy for our day.* 99

I challenge women and girls of all ages worldwide to look in the mirror and say, "Good Morning, Gorgeous," whether they feel like it or not. I am challenging you to start to change your morning routine by finding *one* thing you like about yourself each morning. You truly have to learn to love yourself and the beauty of your soul inside and out. I can tell you right now that looking at yourself and saying, "Good Morning Gorgeous" is probably going to feel weird. It's OK—let it feel weird. If you practice this habit enough, I am praying that it will start to feel weird when you *don't* think it or say it to yourself. When you wake up and say, "Good Morning Gorgeous," it's not a statement of arrogance, it's a statement of gratitude. You should be grateful for the reflection you see looking back at you and grateful for the opportunity to wake up and start a new day.

After you speak it to yourself, I want you to text, call, e-mail, or say it in person to five other women each day. Pay it forward. I truly want you to watch and be aware of the ripple effect that just sharing those words can have on someone's soul. They will light up the minute you say it to them. Speak those words of encouragement to your friends, your daughters, your coworkers, and even total strangers. Negative is normal, and it is up to us to start to change that—it must begin with ourselves.

I receive phone calls, texts, and e-mails daily giving me updates on the effects of the Good Morning Gorgeous campaign. It has been hilarious at times to hear the responses others get when they share this message with family and friends. Here is one of my favorite stories from an audience member:

> One day I walked into the office around eight thirty a.m. I decided to send the entire team a text: "Good Morning Gorgeous, have a great day." Instantly, I started receiving messages asking me if I had been drinking that early in the morning. I just laughed out loud.

As funny as this story is, it proves to me what I have felt for a long time: negative is normal. We expect to hear negative things. So few people see anything "gorgeous" about themselves; hearing that phrase makes them uncomfortable. You are now part of this Good Morning Gorgeous campaign to empower yourself and others to find the light from within and let it shine.

I will tell you it's not easy, even when it's a habit that has been established for years. When I share messages with my audiences that are important to me, I always want them to leave my presentations with a reminder of that message. A few years ago, I created a postcard to remind everyone to start their day with Good Morning Gorgeous and to remind them of my definition of beauty, which is an acronym. It says, "Good Morning Gorgeous," with my acronym for beauty:

Believe in Yourself

Expect the Best

Aspire to Greatness

Utilize Your Gifts

Trust Your Heart

YOU Are Gorgeous!

I have also created hot pink rubber bracelets that say *Good Morning Gorgeous*. If you want a copy of the postcard or a bracelet, simply e-mail us at Dale@winnersbychoice.com and we will mail them out to you.

❝*Good Morning Gorgeous!*❞

Name Your Nag

As I said earlier, women often go on a verbal assault of themselves before they ever leave the bathroom in the morning and many times throughout the day. Whether that assault is quietly inside their head or out loud, they are telling themselves everything they cannot stand about their physical appearance. Also, they tell themselves how tired they are, how stressed they are, and everything else that goes hand in hand with our lives today in the twenty-first century. Your internal nag is sitting in her judgment seat before your first cup of coffee.

I want you to think about your routine. Do you get up and look in the mirror daily and recognize the great things about yourself? Do you see the sparkle in your eyes, the beauty of your face, the color of your hair? Do you see the gorgeous good in you? Do you look in the mirror with gratitude that you are alive to see another day? Or does your internal nag show up and start pointing out all of your flaws instantly? I know that answer, because I have asked those questions a thousand times, and it is a rare occasion when someone will tell me they look in the mirror and see good things. In fact, the negative is so automatic, and it happens so often, that many women don't even realize they are doing it until I point it out to them. It has become their "normal."

Before we move on to counteract this barrage of negativity, I want to stop and encourage you to "name your nag." Psychologist Tamar Chansky says, "Naming it something goofy adds a bit of levity, which helps break through the emotional hold that anxiety has on you. Over time, this short circuits the whole anxious cycle."

Yes, you are going to name the negative voice in your head. It can be your "Inner Gremlin," your "Negative Neva," your "Daphne Downer," or just a name you choose that you can identify with.

Please take a moment and give your negative voice a name. We have left several spaces so you can try out several names for your negative voice. Give it a name you can speak back to when you start hearing that negative message. For instance, "No, Doubting Dale, I am not accepting that message."

_____

_____

_____

_____

_____

_____

The old voice that I identified with for so long was my Doubting Dale. I doubted everything about myself and my ability for so long. I finally had to accept that Doubting Dale could only speak up and be heard if I gave her the floor. The negative voice in our head can only rule our life and our attitude if we choose to allow it to take control; you have to recognize and acknowledge that you have given that voice power.

Once you start to identify the negative voice and all of the messages you are getting from that inner dialogue, you can begin to work on overriding that voice. How do you override it? You replace those discouraging messages with messages that empower and encourage. It is time to start the repetition with positive messages instead of negative ones. Jim Carrey said in his interview with Oprah that he made his affirmations every night. He repeated them over and over. It takes repetition to change anything in our lives, especially to change our internal chatter.

Now is your chance to do a bit of self-reflection. I encourage you to allow yourself to take that journey and look within for a moment before continuing. I want you to write down your three best qualities both inside and out—can you do it right now?

_____

_____

_____

_____

_____

_____

_____

Can you tell me, without hesitation, what you really like about yourself?

_____

_____

_____

_____

_____

_____

_____

If I asked you to tell me instantly the three best words that describe you, what would they be?

_____

_____

_____

_____

_____

_____

_____

Were any of the above questions difficult? Were you able to answer them, or did you skip over one, two, or maybe all three?

I have shared this personal empowerment exercise many times, and anytime I ask my audience to write down their best physical qualities, I see hesitation. I speak to mostly adult groups, but occasionally I am fortunate enough to speak to teenagers. In a recent workshop with teenage girls, I asked them the same questions. I asked them to identify what they really liked about themselves. Just like the adults, they struggled with finding anything they liked about themselves. They were quick to point out what they didn't like. I think I was shocked at first because I have been on this self-growth path for so long. But honestly, I don't know why I was shocked. I was the same way as a teenager.

There was nothing I liked about my physical appearance. In fact, I hear horror stories from my friends who are raising daughters and how they have had their self-esteem damaged because of the negative messages they get from other girls. I hear the stories of girls suffering through bullying at every age. The effect is so much more powerful now due to social media. These young women are subjected to ridicule at a level my generation never experienced.

If we as women, mentors, mothers, teachers, and friends want to change this for generations of young women, we have to not only teach them with our words but also model the behavior in front of them. We have to light and lead the way for them. They are listening to us and learning from us. Let's make sure that what they are learning is empowering them and teaching them to be proud of who they are at any age. The way they hear us describe ourselves and talk about ourselves has a ripple effect.

We have to individually become accountable to ourselves. How can you be accountable for the things you are saying to your soul? You listen. I mean, you *really* listen to yourself. Pay attention to the thoughts and the words you are using to describe yourself and your life. The first step to change in any area of your life is acknowledgment. You can never change what you do not acknowledge.

66 *The most important conversations, briefings, meetings, and lectures you will ever have will be those you hold with yourself in the privacy of your own mind.* 99

Denis Waitley

If you don't like how you feel about yourself or how your life is going, look at the seeds you have planted in your soul. You are the *only* person who can quiet that voice from within. Everyone in the world could tell you that you are talented, gifted, and beautiful; if your inner dialogue is running daily with the opposite message, it will win! It will become your self-fulfilling prophecy. There is an

African proverb that says it best: "When there is no enemy within, the enemies outside cannot hurt you." That one sentence is so powerful. I urge you to write it down and read it often!

Start now to write down the phrases that have wrapped around you for a long time and limited you. What are the phrases and descriptions you have used about yourself for years? Are they really true, or have you just made them your truth? Maybe it's one of these phrases: "I'm too old to follow my dream." "I don't have the time to write my book." "There is nothing special about me."

Write down the phrases that have limited you:

_____

_____

_____

_____

_____

_____

_____

If someone really followed you around for years with this same abusive message, wouldn't you call the police and file a harassment charge? Yet we allow those messages to show up over and over again. Most of the time those limiting messages are running rampant because you're either analyzing the past, worrying about the future, or caught up in the busyness of life. We are rarely 100 percent engaged in the present moment; it is only in the present moment that we can separate from the voice in our head.

Write down a positive phrase to replace each of your limiting phrases. It could read like this: "Because I am alive, it's not too late to follow my dreams."

_____

_____

_____

_____

_____

_____

_____

_____

You have to yank this weed of negativity out by the root and replace it with words of power that will help you grow and flourish. You must put yourself on a "negativity fast." Give up the negativity for a few days, then a week, then a month, and eventually give it up completely.

I am often asked for ideas to help change the negative language habit. Here is a fun challenge that you can even do with your family or a friend. It's simply a fun and simple way to reward yourself as you start to change your patterns. When Nick was small, we always made a game out of staying positive, and I promise you that he would let me know if I was using negative words. So here is the idea: each time you are aware of a positive, empowering thought you think about yourself, put something in a jar. You could get a roll of quarters or pennies and put them next to the jar. I did this as a workout goal. I decorated a mason jar with empowering words, and I took monopoly money, and each time I worked out I dropped a dollar in my workout jar. It was so encouraging to see that jar start to fill up.

When I filled the jar, I rewarded myself with something fun. You could have a competition with your family, your friends, and your kids and call it the Empowerment Jar. If you use the play money, have each person write down the empowering word they thought about themselves on the money as it goes in the jar. When the jars are filled, then you reward yourself with a positive action and start a new jar.

If you take this challenge or implement any challenge to start changing the negative to positive, it will not be easy, and it will be a test. Even though it's not easy, I can promise you it will be worth it. I have been truly working on this change for more than twenty-five years, and it's still not easy. It seems to be harder for me when I am really tired.

Recently, after being on the road for over a week with very little sleep, I flew across country to speak for the contestants and to host the Mrs. United States Pageant in Las Vegas. After a six-hour flight, I landed in Vegas very early in the morning, jetlagged and exhausted. I didn't feel great, and I sure didn't feel like I looked great. I caught myself in the middle of an internal verbal assault about how tired I looked and how bad I looked. I was tired, and my internal nag took full advantage.

That negative voice started shouting in my soul things like this: "Really, you're going to speak to *beauty contestants,* but you look like you've been up three weeks without sleep. How can you teach them to say *Good Morning Gorgeous* when you sure can't do it?" Trust me, even though I know better, I was in full-out personal assault. It's *not* easy, even when it's been part of your life for decades. I wasn't just saying it to myself; I was practically in tears on the phone with my manager. He quickly and kindly reminded me of the messages I believe and teach and reminded me that I was there to inspire; it was my exhaustion that was telling me lies.

It's important to have people who will gently remind you of your truth when you can't remember it yourself. I teach this almost daily, and at times it's still hard for me. It was hard for me when I was so exhausted. But I stopped the negative assault and went and shared my message. And when I saw the pictures that we took that day, I realized that I didn't look as tired as I'd thought I did. My spirit of joy and dealing hope to these incredible women overshadowed any bags under my eyes.

Most of the time I can catch myself focusing on something, becoming a little negative, and I will stop. I get myself in the present moment and change what I say. When you change what you say to yourself, then you will start to change what you see. You will be amazed that if you stop focusing on the little lines around your eyes, eventually you won't see them anymore. You will stop seeing the lines and remember the laughter that put those beautiful reminders on your face.

One of the quotes that has impacted me so much is a quote by speaker and author Mike Murdock that simply says, "Never complain about what you permit." Honestly, that was hard for me when I first read it years ago. But I understand it more every day. I couldn't complain about being exhausted, because I "permitted" everything I added to my schedule. If you are constantly complaining and talking negatively about your body because you don't like something about your body, but you are unwilling to change it, I encourage you to think about this quote. If you aren't going to change it, then you don't earn the right to complain about it.

Your friends and family get sick of hearing about all the things you don't like in your life, yet you are unwilling to make the changes that are necessary. Again, I know these principles, and yet recently someone reminded me of how much I talk about my crazy schedule. I permit that schedule, and I love what I do, so I am now aware of how I describe it to others. It's up to *me*! As much as I would like to, I can't hire a personal trainer to do my sit-ups for me, or do my cardio or my lunges for me. You can't hire someone to exercise for you, and you can't hire someone to speak positively for you. It is up to you! Your personal development is up to you and no one else.

66*Never complain about what you permit.***99**

Do the Work

Yes, trust me—changing these messages and continuing to change them on a daily basis is work. It is not a one-time decision. It is a *daily* decision. If you want to make your life better, you have to have personal, self-motivation to do the hard work on yourself. Does this come naturally? No, not usually. We are surrounded by a world of negativity. There are messages daily showing us what we should be or what we should look like. We have to get to a place in our lives where those images don't affect our personal image. We have to be strong in who we are and who God created us to be.

You are a special and fabulous person. God made you—only you—to be who you are. Don't cheat the world of your beauty, your brilliance, and your love because of your negative view of yourself. Someone needs to be inspired by you. Someone needs you to accept who you are and share that with the world. You need to know that even though I can't see you, I know you are special, and in less than a minute I could find your positive qualities.

If your assault has gone on your entire life and you can't find one thing you like about yourself, ask someone you trust to say one thing they like about you. Now, you may get a friend or two who giggles and gives you the generic, "You're a good person," and though this may be the truth, you need a bit more than that. Tell them you are doing a personal inventory, and you would like their feedback on you. Offer to do the same thing for them. Again, this isn't going to be easy. It's not easy to ask someone to do this for you.

You have an excuse now; you're reading this book, and you can tell them you want to practice this exercise. I encourage you to ask your trusted person to write them down or text them to you so you can refer to them often. In times of difficulty and stress, it helps to be able to go back and read positive things that others see in us. I think you will also be surprised when you ask for this input that you may hear positive things about yourself that you have never considered. I also encourage you to accept the positive thoughts that are given to you, even if you don't believe them about yourself. If you ask for the input, then be gracious in receiving it.

> 66 *There is nothing more rare, nor more beautiful, than a woman being unapologetically herself; comfortable in her perfect imperfection. To me, that is the true essence of beauty.* 99

> STEVE MAROBOLI

Change the Channel

How many times are you in the car with your kids listening to either music or talk radio and they start screaming for you to change the channel? They don't like what they are hearing, and therefore they want it changed. We all do that. We see something on television that makes us uncomfortable; we change the channel. We have to apply this same technique to our lives if we are going to wage war with negativity. If you have the habit of negativity in your life, or even if you don't, there are ways we can change our lives by making minor changes. The little changes will render big results. The big decisions in your life start with little decisions.

Repetition is a powerful *change the channel* skill. It is how we learn everything in our lives. We learn to walk and drive a car, and we learn messages all through repetition. Think about music. Can you hear a song on the radio from your high school or college days and still sing every word? Of course you can. Is it because you sat down with the lyrics and memorized every word? Of course not; it is because you heard those words over and over and over again.

Subconscious repetition—changing the channel was at play. That skill also applies to negative messages that we hear daily, both from outside sources and the internal dialogue we repeat daily. We want to live positive and productive lives, yet so many times we are only tuned in to the draining and destructive messages. The first step to changing the fuel in our internal batteries from negative to positive is recognizing the need for change.

If you recognize the need for change in your life, then you have to make the time for change. The negative messages are more powerful because of all the repetition. When I started to focus on change from the inside out, I had to learn ways I could repeat all of the positive messages I was trying to instill in my life. One of the things I did years ago was loaded my car with positive CDs that I could listen to over and over again.

The late, great, transformational speaker Jim Rohn said, "Turn your car into a rolling university." I remember how much I loved that when I heard it. Listening to empowerment information was like going to class in the school of life—the University of Life. I started turning off the radio and putting down my phone and using whatever time I had in the car to fuel my soul—to go to class. Instead of just socializing on the phone while I was driving, I started learning. Now, even if you don't have a CD player, you can turn on a podcast or satellite radio.

I love to listen to all of my music on Spotify, but I also balance listening to music with great teachers who have a great impact on my life. It's been proven that you need to hear something seven times before it sinks into your soul. Think about that—seven times. I have some of the same CDs in my car that I have been listening to for years, because each time I hear them, I learn something new. You will need to hear the messages that I am teaching in this book more than once if you want them to work in your life. I encourage you to refer to this book often and make notes, use different colored highlighters to mark your journey. Date each time you highlight in a different color. When you refer to something you have read before, you will see how much you have grown.

I remember the first motivational, positive thinking book I ever read, *Seeds of Greatness* by Dr. Denis Waitley. I am sure one of the reasons this book spoke to me was because he talked about planting and harvesting. He asked readers to think about what we were planting and harvesting and how we could expect to harvest well when we were planting bad. Wow. I knew my daddy did not plant corn and expect cotton to come up. If he planted corn, he got corn. It instantly hit me that all I had ever planted in my soul was seeds of doubt, fear, and negativity. Dr. Waitley stated that each one of us has seeds of greatness inside of us, waiting to be nurtured and cultivated. He went on to explain in his book *The 10 Seeds* that can lead to a productive, fulfilling life.

I remember this quote that jumped off the page for me: "It's not what you are that holds you back, it's what you think you're not." Wow, all I had ever thought about and focused on was what I thought I wasn't. Those thoughts had directed my life. That book truly changed my life; it started my journey into personal growth and started to help me change the way I was thinking. If you want to add a book to your library that can change your life, go grab a copy of *Seeds of Greatness,* written more than thirty years ago.

If you had told me growing up that one day I would write a book with the title *Good Morning Gorgeous* or that I would have a career as a professional speaker, I would have thought you had lost your mind. I was shy, scared, and insecure, and I didn't understand any of the life principles I am sharing with you in this book. The principles I now live by everyday were not part of my life. I was unsure about everything. My mind was running full speed with the seeds I had planted deep in my soul, I was watering those thoughts with repetition and focus, and those thoughts grew and became the messages that I believed.

Those messages said, "You aren't talented enough, smart enough, pretty enough, or athletic enough." I focused on all the things that I thought I *wasn't* and gave more and more fuel to those ideas. The more I allowed that voice to speak to me, the louder, more powerful, and more convincing it became.

At that time in my life, I was surrounded by friends who were doing great things in their lives. I felt like I was standing in the shadows, watching other people follow their dreams and use their greatest talents, and I had nothing to offer. I had told myself over and over that I didn't have any real talent; I had told myself that I wasn't pretty enough; I had told myself that I wasn't special in any way. No one had told me those things; I was the author of all of those messages.

That dialogue I was using, the message I was giving to my soul, started to totally distort what I saw in the mirror. As I think back now, I realize that my life was feeling out of control, and I began to convince myself that even if I couldn't be "enough" in all of those areas, I could be "skinny enough." I also see now that because I was surrounded by people who were doing great things, I felt invisible. I truly don't remember making the choice, but I decided there was one thing I could do, and that was to be skinnier. I am five feet eight inches tall and have never been overweight.

Feeling powerless at that time in my life led me to take control over the thing I knew I could control: the number on the scale. In college, I had weighed a healthy 125 pounds, and within two years I watched the scales drop down to 103 pounds. Not only did I lose the weight, but I was also losing myself. I was working my dream job at the time. I had a friend who was a former Miss America. She had a book deal and a recording contract, and she was speaking and singing all over the country. She invited me to move to Nashville to work as her booking agent and road manager. I loved my job but didn't realize I was losing myself. I couldn't see what I was doing to myself.

It was my friend who told me very lovingly but sternly that if I didn't get it under control, she would check me into a hospital. I valued her judgment as a boss and as a friend. I looked up to her so much. I saw the fear and concern on her face, and it was truly my wakeup call. I am not sure that I believed her at the time, but I loved my job, and I didn't want to disappoint her.

I remember the day I looked at my body in the mirror and saw every rib; it scared me. I took a long look at myself and finally saw what others were seeing. I looked like I had been starving myself. That was in the early '80s. My earliest recollection of anorexia was when Karen Carpenter had died from heart failure as a result of a complication of her eating disorder. I know many of you have no idea who that is, but she was one of the most amazing singers this world has ever known. She had starved herself to death. I know exactly where I was when I heard that story. I was stunned when I saw the pictures of Karen Carpenter and realized that my body was starting to look very similar to hers. She went from 145 pounds to 120 pounds and then continued the spiral down to 90 pounds. It had never occurred to me that being so thin and underweight could have other health complications.

It truly made me stop and start honestly asking myself tough questions. Could this happen to me? What had I done to myself and why? Why couldn't I see what everyone had been telling me for years? Thank the dear Lord above that I truly took a good look at my life and what I was doing, and I started that inner journey of discovery and recovery. I was standing on the verge of a serious eating disorder and other health problems, and I knew that I had to make some drastic changes in my life. I knew that it wasn't just my physical body I needed to take care of, but it was my mind I had to change. So I did. I made a choice to change from the inside out.

Even now, thirty years later, when my life feels a little out of control, I will see a number on the scale and my instant reaction is "I can change that." The difference now is that it's only an instant, and all the work I have done from the inside out, and all the books I have read, and all the words and messages on CDs I have fed into my soul overtake that one moment; I go forward with my day.

What is your challenge? What is your inner voice saying to you? What damage have you done to your soul, your spirit, and maybe even your body because of the garbage you have allowed to run rampant in your mind? I am going to ask you to stop right now on this page and write down the messages your inner voice has been telling you for years. Think about what you have told yourself and how it has affected you. You can't expect to eat horrible food every day and be healthy. You also can't expect to put harmful, hurtful messages into your soul and have a healthy mindset. The good news is that regardless of where you have been you can *change the channel,* starting today. The remote is in your hand, and it is your choice.

What is your challenge? What is your inner voice saying to you?

_____

_____

_____

_____

_____

_____

_____

I also challenge you to surround yourself with people who lift you higher. We are all going to have down days, and we need someone else to believe in us when we can't believe in ourselves. Find someone to tell you the truth, as my friend Cheryl did for me. Find at least one person in your life who will do that for you and be that person for someone. Let's be the light for each other and help each other when we can't seem to help ourselves.

66 *Nothing makes a woman more beautiful than the belief she is beautiful.* 99

SOPHIA LOREN

66 *Tell me how a person judges his or her self-esteem and I will tell you how that person operates at work, in love, in parenting, in every important aspect of existence—and how high he or she is likely to rise. The reputation you have with yourself—your self-esteem—is the single most important factor for a fulfilling life.* 99

NATHANIEL BRANDEN

Take Aways

_____

_____

_____

_____

_____

_____

_____

_____

_____

_____

_____

_____

_____

_____

_____

_____

_____

_____

Take Aways

_____

_____

_____

_____

_____

_____

_____

_____

_____

_____

_____

_____

_____

_____

_____

_____

_____

_____

_____

Knowing yourself is the beginning of all wisdom.

ARISTOTLE

GIFT FOUR

Find Yourself—Know Yourself

#GMG

Know Yourself

I can honestly say that all the years I was battling low self-esteem, it was because I had no idea who I was and I didn't know how to find out. "Who are you?" What a question. I don't know why, but when I hear that question, I instantly think of Dorothy in *The Wizard of Oz,* one of my favorite movies of all time. I fell in love with it again when Nick was little because we watched it a million times. Well, not a million, but if you are a mother with small children, you know what I mean. It feels like a million, because they want to watch the same movie over and over again. Kids can usually tell you everything about the movie they love, because at a young age they are already using the power of repetition as a learning tool.

Do you remember when Dorothy landed among the munchkins, and they kept saying, "Are you a good witch or a bad witch?" She just kept saying, "I am Dorothy Gale from Kansas." One of the reasons I love this movie is that it is truly about knowing who you are and what you stand for, following your dreams, and surrounding yourself with positive people who encourage you.

If you ever go back and take a close look at that movie, there are so many life and leadership principles scattered throughout every part of the movie. Dorothy and her pals showed us all that part of knowing who you are is also facing your fear of what you think you are not. This ageless movie shows us three simple but powerful principles through the characters that can encourage all of us. We learned if you use your brain and apply some knowledge, connect to your heart, and face your fear with courage, you can find your way to the desires of your heart. It sounds so simple, doesn't it? Well, it may be simple, but it's not easy, and it all starts with digging deep and knowing who you truly are.

So I am asking you, *who are you?* Have you ever stopped to think about the answer to that question? *Who are you?* I don't think it's a question that we often get asked. We get asked our name, what we "do," if we are married or single, if we have kids or not, but we rarely get this very strong question. So I am going to be the one to ask you.

I encourage you to pause right now and think about that question. Answer the question as if you and I were talking in person. What would you say? Would you tell me where you lived or if you were married or single or where you worked? I am willing to guess that you would. But is that who you really are? Those details may describe us—our titles and our lives—but are they really *who we are?* We seem to always define ourselves by our marital status, whether we have children, where we live, or where we work. We define ourselves by *what* we do, not *who* we are. The other labels that we put on ourselves sound like this: I am tired, worn out, guilty, stressed, and exhausted.

I rarely hear *I am a wonderful, inspiring, educated, sensational woman who seeks to make a difference daily* or anything close to that description. But my hope is that after reading this chapter, that will change. I will tell you when I first started asking that question to my audiences, I realized I also had not answered it. So I took the time to answer that question, and here is my answer, "I am an unapologetic optimist who has a passion and a life purpose to deal hope around the world and to make a difference daily."

Who are you *really,* from the inside out? What makes you unique, special, and different? What truly makes your heart sing with happiness? What is your life's purpose? What sets you apart, and what makes you different? If anyone had asked me that question until I was in my thirties, I would not have had an answer. Our identity, how we view ourselves, comes from our *self-image.* I know we have all heard that phrase so many times, but do we even know what it really means? Self-image is how we value ourselves—how we see ourselves. It is how we perceive our value to the world and how valuable we think we are to others. Self-image affects our trust in others, our relationships, our work, how or if we follow our dreams—nearly every part of our lives. Positive self-esteem gives us the strength and flexibility to take charge of our lives and grow from our mistakes without the fear of rejection.

It seems we spend the first twenty years of our lives trying to fit in and be accepted. We want to be popular, accepted, and one of the gang. We want to be chosen. We want to be valued. One of the first interesting and dramatic attempts at acceptance in my life was trying to get elected as cheerleader at Eupora High School. Eupora High School where my graduating class had eighty-two students. Yes, I said *dramatic,* because at fifteen it was dramatic, everything at fifteen is dramatic. Looking back now, I realize that I felt if I could be elected cheerleader it meant that I was OK; I was accepted and valued. Being a cheerleader during those days was just a popular vote by the students, not an athletic event like it is now. The only requirement to be a cheerleader was to be popular. I was a shy, awkward, insecure teenager who lived out in the country. I wasn't popular, I didn't have a boyfriend, and I didn't live "in town." I think I felt if I could win that election and be a cheerleader, then those feelings would change. I would be accepted and valuable.

❝Positive self-esteem gives us the strength and flexibility to take charge of our lives and grow from our mistakes without the fear of rejection.❞

As you can imagine, I didn't win that election. In fact, I lost by just a few votes, and my first real-life heartbreak was not because I lost a boyfriend but because I lost the cheerleader election. But months later, as I was still getting over that loss, one of the girls dropped out and I got to take her place. I was a cheerleader. But it had never occurred to me that cheerleaders had a job—it wasn't just a title. I still remember the day the head cheerleader told me that if I didn't get over my insecurity and start talking to the students and the football players I would be dismissed from the squad. I can tell you that the thought of losing my spot on the cheerleading squad was much more painful than the thought of talking to people, especially to the football players. So I took action, faced my fear, started facing my insecurity, and remained a cheerleader throughout high school. I was even head cheerleader my senior year. It was years later that I understood that we will do more to avoid pain than to gain pleasure. I faced some of my biggest fears to avoid the pain of not remaining on the squad.

As we get older, I think we all look back from time to time and wish we could have really understood the value of the lesson at the time it was happening. Of course, the lesson for me was that becoming a cheerleader did not make me fit in or feel valuable. It was the experience—what I learned through that experience and who I became through that experience—that changed me. The more I stepped out of my shadow of doubt and accepted myself, the more I was accepted by others. I didn't realize it then, but facing defeat, feeling heartbroken, and finding ways to move past those emotions were part of the life lessons that were so valuable.

We are all going to feel bad about ourselves from time to time, but when that feeling hangs around and it's with you all the time, do some investigating and see if your self-esteem needs some attention. During my teenage and college years, I had the classic signs of someone dealing with low self-esteem. I had started to face the shyness, but I had not faced the low self-esteem. I was very critical of myself; I was always comparing myself to other people. I focused on the negatives and constantly spoke negatively, never accepting any compliments. I know that my low self-esteem was the contributor to my brush with an eating disorder. If you start to see these behaviors creeping into your life, then it's time to pause, take a look within, and give your self-esteem some love and attention.

Like I said earlier, I feel that if we spend the first twenty years trying to be accepted and fit in, then we spend the next twenty to forty years trying to separate ourselves from the pack, truly trying to identify who we are and discover our authentic self. Discover your authentic self, know who you are—we are never taught how to do that. We are not taught how to make that personal discovery. I don't know about you, but there wasn't an Authentic Self 101 class in my high school or college that would guide me through that process of discovering who I was. If there had been, this girly girl who loves high heels and does not have an athletic bone in her body would not have ended up in the physical education department at Mississippi State getting a BS degree. You know that is a bachelor of science degree, but I can say with a smile on my face that the slang definition of BS is totally appropriate here. You will read more about that adventure later in this chapter.

I am happy to say things have changed over the years and I know at least one college campus that is helping students on their personal path. My friend Dr. Nido Qubein is the president of High Point University, and he has made it mandatory for all first-year students to take his Life Skills class to help them learn and understand the skills necessary for all areas of life. They are taught how to build their self-esteem, how to set goals for themselves, and how to be great leaders, plus so much more. I was blown away when I heard Dr.

Qubein talk about this class and all the aspects of it. They are truly teaching these students to know who they are and how to be their personal best in all phases of their lives.

I was touring High Point University with some of my other speaker friends, and Nido told us about this class. Honestly, I wanted to enroll in High Point at that moment just to take that class. I love that the first paragraph in the course description is about self-esteem. It is so powerful—I want you to read the first course objective. It says, "to teach you how to gain a positive self-esteem. Positive self-esteem can give you the character to face any obstacle that stands in your way. With high self-esteem, you can meet the most disappointing and discouraging situations with faith, hope, and courage." Isn't that awesome? Because the course has been such a hit with students and parents, a companion course for seniors is now being offered. If you don't know about High Point University, check it out. It's a remarkable story and a remarkable university led by a remarkable man, Nido Qubein, who has changed the path of High Point.

So, if you are not a student at High Point signed up for a Life Skills class, how do you build your self-esteem, discover who you are, embrace it, and apply it to your life? How do you find that personal self-acceptance? I am going to help you with that, but first we must understand this path of personal discovery.

The road to total self-acceptance, positive self-esteem, and identity is not an easy journey. It is also a road that does not have an end destination. It will be a lifelong journey. If you truly get committed to knowing yourself, accepting yourself, and building your self-esteem, it will get easier. When you are determined to create and sustain a higher self-esteem—even when your value gets challenged—you won't let it affect you as long. You will notice it, acknowledge it, and let it go.

Regardless of where you feel your self-esteem is right now on a scale from one to ten, I promise you that it can get better. This is one place in our lives where there is the opportunity for constant and never-ending improvement. I believe that building your self-esteem is like going to the gym to build your muscles. You have to work at it. Your self-esteem muscle needs work, and it takes awareness and effort. It is a life skill and a skill that you will continue to work on daily. My goal for you is that when you begin to apply these thoughts, principles, and ideas, you will be able to walk into any room, any situation, with confidence in who you are, and the only validation you will need to make that your reality is yours. You will know that the person whose opinion matters the most is yours. Building this kind of internal strength, this internal image of value, will not just be work, it will be hard work. Just like professional athletes have to go to the gym every day to work on their skills, we have to go to work every day to work on our mindset. To be all you were created to be, to accomplish the goals and dreams you want to accomplish, to achieve personal excellence you have to build the most important thing, *you*!

We have already covered several of the skills that are critical in helping you build your self-esteem. One of the biggest keys is the self-talk we explored in the previous chapter. That internal voice of authority is either going to build you up or take you down. If you are tearing yourself down from within, you will be on the constant search for someone else to make you feel better about yourself.

I see so many women battle that desperate search for validation—always looking outside of themselves for someone, and many times some man, to give them the words they need to feel valuable, beautiful, smart, and special. Of course, it is great and empowering to hear words of affirmation from others, but we can't wait on those words to create our value.

I want you to hear me when I tell you that *no one* can give you your self-worth and *no one* can take it away. If you do not feel valuable from within, it doesn't matter how many words you hear telling you that you are special, smart, beautiful, unique, or any other positive word, it will never be enough. That void can only be filled from within. It's a message you will hear from me more than once in this book. You may get sick of hearing it, but I hope I say it so much that you won't forget it. I hope I reinforce the message to you in the pages of this book what it took me *decades* to learn. I can tell you that I am still learning. I hope my growth path can shorten your growth path. If the fact that I have walked through and learned on my journey can help you find that truth in a shorter amount of time, that will be one of the greatest accomplishments of my life.

> ❝ *No one can give you your self-worth and no one can take it away.* ❞

Your self-esteem requires sole/soul ownership. No one can steal your self-esteem, and no one can give it to you. If your self-esteem is strong, even if someone says something or does something that hurts your feelings, it doesn't change your value or view of yourself. You simply acknowledge your feelings and move on. If you are continually looking for someone else or some accomplishment to make you feel good about yourself, you will be in a search your entire life. No one can you give you the belief that you must give to yourself.

Self-talk is the first key in building our self-esteem, and the second key is giving up the comparison game. It's a critical to stop comparing yourself if you want to build your self-esteem to a stronger level. I love this quote: "Don't compare your first chapter to someone else's chapter 20." Isn't that great?

If you are comparing your singing ability to someone else's, you don't know how long they have worked at their craft. If you are comparing your talent, your physical ability, or your appearance to anyone else's, I challenge you to stop. Stop looking at who they are or what they are doing and get your focus on taking 100 percent responsibility for yourself and your life. If you are comparing yourself to someone in the public eye, you are only seeing what they are being rewarded for in public. You are the not seeing the years of work, defeat, dedication, and struggle it took them to get there. Of course, I believe in having mentors and learning from other people. But there is a *big* difference between comparing and learning. When you are learning, you are asking questions and seeking information that will help you grow. If you are comparing yourself, you are tearing yourself down for what you are not. That isn't growth—that is only disappointment. You can feel the difference in your soul, so make sure you are paying attention.

The Power of Five

I remember when I first read about this concept by author Jim Rohn, who I mentioned earlier as the inspiration to turn my car into a "rolling university." He stated that we are the average of the five people that we choose to spend the most time with. I am not talking about family or the people you work with. I am talking about your friends—the people you choose to spend time with. What conversations are you having? Who are you texting and hanging out with?

What did Jim Rohn mean with that statement? He meant that if the five people you spend the most time with are very negative, there is a very good chance you will also adopt that negative mentality. On the other hand, if you spend time with five positive people, then you are more likely to mirror that behavior. If you are around positive people, who are setting goals and following their dreams, you are more likely to have the courage to talk about *your* goals and dreams. I want you to truly think about the people you share most of your time with and ask yourself if they increase you or decrease you. Is your energy elevated or drained? Do they encourage you, or are they telling you why your goals and dreams won't come true? Take a moment and journal your answers in the following spaces.

_____

_____

_____

_____

_____

_____

_____

_____

If anyone is giving advice to you about your life, your goals, or your dreams, I want you to just pause and ask yourself, *Is this someone I should be taking advice from?* If this person is not living the life you want to live—if he or she is not the type of person you want to be—I encourage you not to take that person's advice. Listen and get guidance from people who are living the life you want to live. Get advice from people who know who they are and where they are going in their lives.

> ❝ *When we don't know our internal value, and we are not clear about the direction of our life, it's very easy to accept any message that we are given.* ❞

Your *value* is only for you to decide. I have friends who have been through tremendous verbally abusive situations where a husband or a boyfriend was telling them how worthless and horrible they were. It's so hard not to drink of that poison when it comes from someone you love. But let me be very clear: if a man or anyone else is degrading you, talking down to you, and verbally attacking you, that is *not* loving; that is abuse. It's hard not to take those words and let them be your truth. It's hard to feel valuable when you are hearing the worst possible things you could hear about yourself from someone who is important to you or who was once important to you. There will be people in life who try to use words as a weapon of destruction to your soul. That weapon can only prosper if you give it power and make it *your* truth. Those words only become truth when *you* accept them as your reality. When you stand in your true worth and value, you will instantly reject the words that do not ring true in your soul.

I know that some of you may have been through horrible situations where your very core was shaken. I just want to remind you that no one has the right to talk to you or treat you as if you do not have value. You are worthy of being treated with respect, honor, and kindness. Each of us is responsible for building this place of worth within ourselves and finding our peace from within. When you are at true peace with yourself, then nothing external can shake that peace.

When you know, truly *know*, that God made you a valuable, special person, no one's words or actions can take that from you.

If someone starts to verbally attack you or your character, I urge you—if at all possible—to leave the room and get out of the assault. Imagine yourself with a bulletproof vest wrapped snuggly around your soul, and each word of attack hits you but slides off and doesn't cause you harm. The words and opinions of someone else are like water. All the water in the world can't harm you unless it gets inside of you. All the words in the world can't harm you unless you pick them up and accept them as your truth. As we all learned from the movie, *The Help,* "You is kind. You is smart. You is important!"

A man ending a relationship with you that you believed in will hurt; someone speaking harmful words to you or about you will hurt; someone dissolving a friendship with you will hurt—yet it doesn't have to shake your peace or define who you are. Who you are is not determined by your relationship status, your age, or anything else. Sure, getting older can challenge you, but it doesn't have to steal your peace or create your identity. Your opinion of you is the one that counts the most. Yes, we want to be accepted by others, but being accepted by ourselves *first* is the most critical step. When you *know* who you are, someone's opinion of you will *never* be your reality.

As I travel around the world as a speaker, my audience members often ask questions about discovering their true gifts and talents. It seems that many people struggle to find their true path and are challenged to truly understand their skill set. I know it was a long journey for me. I was in my early thirties when a dear friend recommended I take the Myers-Briggs Type Indicator test. This well-known personality test presents you with many questions and then evaluates your personality profile based on your answers. What an incredible eye-opener that test was for me. I remember the day I took the test. I sat anxiously waiting for the results. When I finally received them and read the long results sheet, I was almost in tears.

It was as if this team of researchers had been spying on me my entire life. My personality type is ENFP. What amazed me was that every characteristic of this personality type is exactly who I am. In a strange way, I felt validated and recognized. For years, I thought I was different and just didn't fit in. I see now that that was more because of my insecurity than my personality. But we are all different, and we should be proud of it.

Still, it seems that we always identify *different* as *strange*. It took me well into my thirties to accept this, be proud of it, and celebrate it. One of the greatest quotes I have ever heard came from one of my best friends. She just happens to be the mother of one of the biggest pop stars in the world, who stood on stage at an awards presentation and stated that his mother had taught him, "If you want to make a difference, you have to be different." How powerful is that? The next time you feel *different,* stop and ask yourself how you can use your uniqueness to make a difference.

Who Do You Think You Are?

I want to share a little more with you about the struggle of my own personal inner journey. I hope that my willingness to be open and share my journey with you will empower you and encourage you, especially if you can relate to my story. For so much of my life, I could look around and see all of the great gifts, talents, and attributes of everyone around me. I could point them out in an instant. But while I was pointing them out, I was also comparing myself to the other people and noticing what I was *not*. Most of my life, I felt there was nothing that I could do that was great or, in my mind, even above average. I could sing a little and play the piano a little; I was a good student but not a great student. I had zero athletic ability, so team sports were out for me.

I could not identify any activity where I felt I was accomplished. I wonder if you have ever felt that way? I was constantly looking at someone else in my world and wishing I had their beauty, their brains, their athletic ability, or their talent. I could not understand why I wasn't a great singer, athlete, or musician. The more I tried to do all of those things, the more frustrated I became because I was average at best. I realize now that the more I focused on what I did not have, the more I missed the gifts I did have. That old saying is true: if you only look at the door that is closed, you will never see the windows that are open. My skill set was a unique one, and one that was mentioned in the personality profile that I discovered. My natural strengths are in speaking and being on stage. My natural strengths are sharing through the written and spoken word, but due to my total lack of self-esteem for so many years, it took me some time to discover these gifts.

In college, I tried out for the lead in a play but was cast in a supporting role. Once again, I came in second place as the default "winner." When I found out I was only cast in a supporting role, I was taken back to the time in my life when I felt like I was a "default" cheerleader. I was so disappointed, but much like with the cheerleader experience, a few weeks passed and the lead dropped out, and I was asked to take over. It was a great opportunity, and I took the lessons I learned from the cheerleading experience and made the most of it. But that negative voice in my head once again reminded me that I wasn't "chosen" and had ended up there by default. Even in the middle of an experience that I loved, I questioned myself and wondered whether I was "good enough," only because of the way it had happened. I allowed that to overshadow the fact that I did a great job and was credited with much of the success of the play. I allowed what I could control, my inner dialogue, to overshadow the joy and success of the event.

What about you? Have you spent wasted time wondering why you weren't gifted in a certain area, or why something happened a certain way? I knew during my time on stage during the college plays that I had found something I truly loved. But because of my fear and my inner voice, I didn't embrace the things that made my soul sing. I didn't pursue a career in journalism or communication. I got a degree in physical education. You read that right. This high-heel wearing, former beauty queen without an athletic bone in her body got a degree in PE. I laughingly tell people I had no business being in any of those classes because the only thing that runs on me is my mouth. I knew deep down in my soul that I wanted to do something that involved being on stage. However, I didn't have the courage to face the truth of what I wanted, because it didn't seem practical. I also didn't trust that I could be talented enough to follow that dream. Also, there weren't any jobs for actresses in North Mississippi, and I had never thought about really leaving that part of the world. I knew I needed to make the "safe" choice and get the education degree, so I did. If I had faced the truth, I would have known I was going against my natural gifts.

I struggled every step of the way with that degree because it went against every natural ability with which God had sent me to this planet. At the time, I was too scared to even voice my dream of being on stage, and so I chose to follow a path that in my head made sense but in my heart felt so wrong. I was hiding. I believe we hide behind so many things. We hide behind making the "safe" choices, we hide behind someone else's opinion, we hide behind the phrase of *I'm too busy,* we hide behind our excuses, and we hide behind our fear. I want you to search your soul and ask yourself if you are hiding. If you are hiding, what have you been hiding from? Are you hiding from your gifts? Are you hiding from your true goals and dreams? I truly believe that what-ever you run from will eventually be exposed to the light.

It's humbling. I now make my living as a speaker, author, and teacher. As I mentioned, it took me until I was in my thirties to finally recognize my true gifts and start to embrace and develop them. I wonder how many people go through life and never find their true identity and self-worth? If this rings true to you, I want you to know that it is never too late to start. One book that changed my life was a book by Louise Hay Louise didn't write her first book until she was in her late fifties. She became a *New York Times* best-selling author, and her books have sold more than 50 million copies around the world in more than thirty languages. It is *never* too late to discover your gifts and pursue them.

If you are struggling to know yourself as I was, I encourage you to investigate taking a personality profile test. There are all types of personality tests out there; MBTI was just the first one I had ever taken. This test listed the best types of professions for my personality type. The best profession for my type included author, teacher, and being on stage—all the things I am doing now. I had just started speaking when I took the test, and I can't describe the joy I felt when I discovered that the career I had fallen in love with was also the right fit for my personality. If you are struggling at all with finding your strengths and gifts, I urge you to take the MBTI personality test or something similar. It's easy and fun. The one I took can be found at www.discoveryourpersonality.com.

Take a Good Look

Getting comfortable in my skin and taking the MBTI test started me on the path of finding my true inner strengths, which I have since not only worked on but developed. I had to step out of that shadow of doubt and truly take the risk of following a very unique and unusual career path. I make my living doing what every one of us as mothers has taught our children not to do: talk to strangers. I make my living every day walking out on a stage and sharing messages that I believe can make a difference. But it also leaves me open to criticism and harsh evaluation. I still cringe at the audience evaluations that corporations send me after my presentations, and sometimes it takes days for me to open them.

When I first started getting those evaluations, even after all the work I had done on my personal development, I would immediately look to see if there were any negative numbers. I now have accepted that my message will not always be on target for 100 percent of my audience, and my job is to step on the stage and share. If one person leaves with one idea that can change his or her life, then my time was well invested. We are not always going to be accepted by everyone.

It took me years to get comfortable with my talent and embrace my strengths. I know many people who are good at so many things. My son, Nick, is amazing at just about anything he does, but just because he is good at something doesn't make it a strength. I know from experience you also have to have a passion for what you are doing. Marcus Buckingham, the author of *Now, Discover Your Strengths,* says it best, "A better definition of a strength is an activity that makes you feel strong. And a weakness is an activity that makes you feel weak. Even if you're good at it, if it drains you, that's a weakness." Marcus recommends writing down the activities that energize you or drain you during a regular week. He goes on to say that once you have determined your strengths, you need to refine and sharpen your skills: "You grow the most, learn the most, develop the most in the areas where you already have some natural advantage."

I have to stay that stepping on a stage and speaking makes me feel strong. It energizes me, and I love seeing the light of enlightenment when I share something that I know has made a difference. I know many people who get totally paralyzed with fear by having to make a presentation. I get asked all the time if I get nervous before I step on stage. For me, it's the opposite: I get so excited and energized because I know it's my strength and I know that the message really can make a difference. When I step on stage, I feel that I am there to give something to my audience, and it takes away any fear I might have.

I encourage you to do the exercise that Marcus suggests. Write down what energizes you and what drains. Start to take inventory, and you will begin to see your strengths emerge. Once I realized that I truly loved speaking, then I started to work on the skill set that would make me a better presenter.

What energizes you, Gorgeous? What drains you?

_____

_____

_____

_____

_____

_____

_____

What Have You Done for *You* Lately?

Do you remember the Janet Jackson song "What Have You Done for Me Lately?" Maybe you feel that your life is filled with people who are constantly asking you that question. As women, it seems that we are consistently doing for others first before we ever get around to having anyone do anything for us or doing anything for ourselves. Don't get me wrong; I think it's a great quality to have as long as we keep it in balance. I love taking care of my family and friends, but we have to remember to also take care of ourselves.

We cater to the needs of so many people and yet we rarely even recognize our needs. I was recently asked this question: "What are you doing for you?" I have to admit it stopped me in my tracks and haunted me all day. I am very grounded in who I am, but I still struggle with taking care of everyone else and not taking good enough care of myself. I realized the other day I have had a massage gift certificate on my desk for over a year and I haven't made the time to use it. Why? It only takes an hour. But taking that one hour for me seems to be such a sacrifice. We women do not sacrifice enough time for ourselves.

My husband, like a lot of men, does not face this issue at all. He rides motorcycles for himself, he plays video games, he is an avid skier, he plays golf, and he is a wine collector. When I am asked what I do for a hobby or what I do for fun, I again have trouble with the question. Why is this? Why is it that we, mainly women, cannot be like men in the aspect of taking *me* time—doing things for ourselves. Think about this for a moment. This is your time of reflection and learning. This is for you! What about you? What is your hobby? What do you do just for you?

I am learning to take time out for myself. This is truly not an easy lesson for me. I have realized that whenever I do something just for me, I catch myself starting to feel guilty. We must realize that guilt is a choice, not an emotion. You *choose* to feel guilty. No one can make you feel guilty without your consent. I encourage you to teach your daughters, through your example, that it is OK to take time out for themselves. If we want to be the best for other people, then we have to also put ourselves on that list. As women, we are constantly running on empty, and it's because we rarely stop to refuel our souls. What fuels your soul? What brings you total joy? What empowers you and energizes you?

_____

_____

_____

_____

_____

_____

_____

_____

I have continued to ask those questions, and I am asking them to myself as I am writing them to you. I am writing down the answers to those questions, and I am making a promise to visit them often, with the hope that you will do the same. Let's make a commitment to each other, through the pages of this book, to put ourselves on the list. We can serve the world, but we also have to feed ourselves.

Who you truly are is a combination of so many things. It's the combination of your natural gifts, the things you have been willing to learn and change, the risks you have taken, the relationships you have built, the lessons you have learned, the dreams you have for the future, and so much more. I challenge you to think outside the box and continue to discover yourself every day. It doesn't matter how young or how old you are. If you are still blessed to be living this life, then you deserve to live it knowing and celebrating your best self.

I want you to truly dig down and discover or rediscover who you truly are. We are all growing and changing, and this is a process that we will be engaged in our entire lives. I am challenging people to let me know what makes them feel gorgeous, and that doesn't just mean your physical being. What makes you feel gorgeous and joyful from the inside out?

Maybe you feel gorgeous and blessed when you bake cookies with your kids, volunteer for a special cause, or use your gifts to their full potential. The thing that makes your eyes sparkle and your skin glow comes from the spark in your soul and your assurance that regardless of how old you are, you know *who* you are. I hope you will complete the sentence below and keep completing it. The more you focus on what makes you feel gorgeous, the more you attract that into your life.

I feel gorgeous when _____

_____

_____

_____

_____

_____

_____

_____

_____

_____

I also want you to have a go-to list of words that describe you and who you are. I want you to list as many positive, descriptive words you can think of and keep them close so you can refer to them when you need to be reminded. I keep mine in a journal that I can refer to often. Here are a few powerful words to get you started: *unique, special, fierce, powerful, brave, gorgeous, authentic, giving, teachable, one of a kind!*

_____

_____

_____

_____

_____

_____

_____

_____

_____

_____

_____

_____

Go back and highlight the words that truly make you feel stronger; put them somewhere you can see them often.

> *There is a fountain of youth: it is your mind, your talents, the creativity you bring to your life and the lives of people you love. When you learn to tap this source, you will truly have defeated age.*
>
> —Sophia Loren

> *To be beautiful means to be yourself. You don't need to be accepted by others. You need to accept yourself.*
>
> —Thich Nhat Hanh

Take Aways

_____

_____

_____

_____

_____

_____

_____

_____

_____

_____

_____

_____

_____

_____

_____

_____

_____

_____

_____

66 Sometimes life is about risking everything for a dream no one can see but you. 99

GIFT FIVE

Uncover Your Dream

#GMG

What's Your Dream?

"Welcome to Hollywood! What's your dream?" Do you remember that line at the end of the movie *Pretty Woman*? It was a guy standing on a sidewalk holding up a sign and asking people about their dreams. I don't remember any other quote from that movie, but I remember that one. Here's a better question, "Welcome to your life—what's your dream?"

I don't know where many people lose this ability to dream along the way, but it sure seems that they do. We come to this planet wide open and ready to dream the biggest dreams. I remember clearly that by the time my son Nick was five, he was already dreaming of being a fireman, driving a big log truck, and even driving a racecar. I am happy to say that thirty-year-old Nick Thomas has never given up his ability to dream. He was fascinated with cars from an early age, and I remember every time we were on the road, we would play the car game. We would see a car coming toward us and have a contest on who could name the type of car first. That love of cars, dreaming of cars, has led Nick to being a racecar driver. He drives a drift car professionally. Nick Thomas (www.NickThomasRacing.com) is still following his dreams and making sure they come true.

Do you remember a time in your life when it was easy to have a goal or a dream? I hope that the answer is a big *yes,* and if it is not, then I hope the words on this page will encourage and motivate you to ignite your fire of belief. I remember as a little girl watching television and dreaming of being an actress. I never voiced that dream out loud because it seemed so ridiculous for a little girl on a farm in Mississippi to dream of being an actress or being on television.

How could that even be possible? It was a dream that I pushed way down in my soul for so many years, but it never really went away. Through the years, as I have learned how to "lean in" to the dreams in my soul, I have watched so many of them come true. I have had to learn and practice every skill I am writing about in this book, and I want you to know that if I have done it, so can you. I went from not being able to voice my dreams to living dreams that are so big that I am constantly in awe. This book you are holding in your hand is a dream come true. Each time I am honored to step on stage in front of an audience and share my message is a dream come true. I have even fulfilled a "secret" childhood dream.

Several years ago, within a span of about two years, I was on national television five different times. I remember sitting in my dressing room when I was getting ready to be a guest expert on the *Dr. Phil Show* and thinking about how far I had come. The shy little girl from a dirt road in Mississippi who was scared even to voice her dream of being on television was about to go live with Dr. Phil in front of millions of people. If anyone had told me when I was in high school or college that I would one day be living the life I live now, fulfilling my dreams, I would not have believed it. My belief system had to catch up to the dreams that were hidden in my soul.

As I have read about and studied big achievers, the people that we all consider extraordinary, I have learned that they are all dreamers. I have read story after story in which these successful people were told their dreams were unrealistic. Many of them were called crazy (at least at the beginning), but they learned to approach life differently than the masses. That is the key—they approach life differently, or they would never have achieved what they achieved. Throughout this chapter, I will share stories of some of the biggest dreamers of all time. Without the willingness of these dreamers of the world, you wouldn't have the coffee you drink (if you are a Starbucks lover). You wouldn't be reading or watching the enchanted life of Harry Potter (thank you, J. K. Rowling). None of us would have ever experienced the magic of the happiest place on earth (thank you, Walt Disney).

> 66 *Sometimes our beliefs need to catch up to the dreams hidden in our souls.* 99

Many times, we hear of someone's success, and we don't stop and think about what their journey toward the fulfillment of that dream must have been. We don't think about how many *no's* they may have heard along the way. We don't think about how many times they possibly doubted that their dream would ever be a reality. We don't think about how many people probably told them they were crazy for chasing an unrealistic dream. It's easy to celebrate the final product, but the journey is where the power is seen. When a dream is anchored in your heart, and it is truly your dream, then the passion of following it, creating it, is part of the joy of the journey. The dream of this book has been in my heart for a long time, and as I told you earlier, it's taken much longer than I had thought. But I can tell you that I have grown and changed from this journey. I have laid it down at times and walked away. There were days I wasn't sure I would pick it back up again. On those days, I would be reminded of the books that have truly changed my life, and I would remind myself that if there is *one sentence* in this book that can encourage you and empower you, then I was being selfish not to work through the tough days and get it in your hands. I truly don't believe easy is an option when we are pursuing things that really make a difference.

Your dreams and goals are your GPS—your *Goal Pursuing System.* When you turn on the GPS on your phone or in your car, you have to enter your "final" destination so the software can figure out your route. How many of us would be literally, totally, and completely lost without our GPS? How many times have I heard people say, "What in the world did we do before navigation?" I know what we did: we had a map! For me, it was a big map—the atlas. We had to plan the route, try to find the route, and calculate how much time it would take us to drive it—and then we hoped and prayed we could navigate that map on the drive. For those of you who have never done that, it's not easy, especially by yourself! Now, we simply listen to a voice telling us where to go after we have programmed in our final destination. She even corrects us if we are not paying attention and go the wrong way. She tells us how many miles; she tells us how long it will take to get there. My maps even show me the delays on the highway. It's awesome. However, at times I think my "navi-girl" is just messing with me to see if I am paying attention. I end up on some strange road that I know is not the most direct route.

The same concept for our navigation is true for your life direction. If you didn't have a map or GPS and you had never been to your destination, you would just be wandering around hoping you would finally arrive. I believe our lives are the same way; you will just be wandering around until you truly set your course and your destination. Unfortunately, we don't have the "navi-girl" telling us how long it will take us to get to our desired destination in life.

When you begin to program your journey in your soul, it's important to remember that your dreams have to be your dreams and only your dreams. Many times, I have spoken with students who have been talked into the perfect major in college because it was a good choice, but their heart and their passion was totally somewhere else. If you have a dream that is unusual and you share that dream, you may get a lot of feedback about it. I just need to remind you that someone else's opinion of you and your dreams is none of your business. I remember the first time I heard that from another speaker. I had to think about it. When I let those words truly sink in, I realized how powerful they were. I am not saying that you don't seek counsel from people you trust and gather all the wisdom that you can, but I am saying that if your dream seems unrealistic to someone else, you can respect their opinion but you aren't required to follow it. More dreams have never seen the light of day because the opinion of someone else took power over the dream. The dream never got a chance to survive. One person shared his or her doubt that you could make that dream a reality, and then the doubt drowned the dream. In fact, I read recently that there are two kinds of business: your business and none of your business. And again, what someone thinks about your life path is none of your business.

The basic rule for success is we have to take 100 percent responsibility for our life choices. If we choose to allow someone else's ideas to direct our lives, we can't blame them—we made the choice. In every phase and every area of our lives, we have to continue to remind ourselves that we are where we are and who we are based on our choices. It is our choices and not our circumstances that are the catalyst to change all of our lives. You have made the individual choices and decisions that have gotten you to your current place in life, and at any moment you can make a different decision. If you want to have a different life, it is totally up to you to make the choices and decisions today that will eventually get you there. I had to take total responsibility that I had made the choice" to get a degree in physical education because it seemed like the right thing to do.

> 66 *The basic rule for success is we have to take*
> *100 percent responsibility for our life choices.* 99

When I realized it was not the right path for me, I had to make choices to start moving my life in a different direction. I knew that many people would not understand why I would spend four years going to college to get a degree I would never use. Well, I tell them now that even though I have never coached a day in my life on a basketball court, I am now coaching for life around the world. So, I laughingly tell people I am using that degree.

There will usually be two types of people in your life—believers and nonbelievers. You will have the people who will encourage you, believe in you, and give you every reason to believe you can follow your dreams. The other group will try to talk you out of your dreams, telling you to be realistic. Usually, they will claim that it is because they care about you and don't want you to get hurt or be disappointed? The truth is you will be more disappointed if you don't try to follow where you feel you are being led. I remember when I decided to enter the Mrs. Tennessee Pageant in my late twenties. I was so excited about it, but I was not prepared for the looks or the questions I got about being in a beauty pageant at this phase of my life. I remember it hurt my feelings at first that I didn't feel supported. I later realized that the people who were questioning me about my choices were just afraid I would be hurt if it didn't turn out the way I wanted it to.

At that point, I had to make the decision as to whether I was going to allow those opinions to keep me from taking the step I wanted to take. I didn't win the first two years, and yes, it's never fun to lose, but I didn't consider it losing. If you learn from any experience in life, then you never really loose. Growth comes from the down moments. When you miss the mark or "fail," consider that your tuition. If you choose to learn instead of lose, it's the tuition for the next step in your life.

I am so glad I decided to follow my heart—my dream—and even though it took longer than I planned, I learned every step of the way. Each time I didn't win the title, I stopped and asked myself if I had done my best; was there anything I could have done differently? The answers were no and yes. I learned to totally trust myself. I knew that I would know when it was time to alter that dream. The final year I competed at Mrs. Tennessee, I knew that, regardless of the outcome, it was my last year. People are going to have an opinion about your life and what you should or shouldn't do. Here is the biggest challenge: you can't be attached to either opinion, positive or negative. Why? Your direction has to come from within your soul. Here is a quote I love that sums it up perfectly: "If you give people the power to feed you, you also give them the power to starve you." Give that some thought!

Until my early twenties, I totally censored my dreams. I lived in a world of *couldn't*. I *couldn't* be on television, I *couldn't* be on stage, and I *couldn't* do any of the things I was drawn to. Why couldn't I? Because I had *decided* that I couldn't. I used every excuse in the world. I lived in the wrong part of the country, I didn't have the talent, I didn't have the time, and the list went on.

Thankfully, little by little, with the power of personal development and changing my brain, as discussed earlier, I began to take the censors off of myself. I began to take responsibility for those excuses. I began to step up and step out into taking the chance to follow my heart. I began to take baby steps toward those dreams. We have to take the censor off our dreams and start to be a kid again. We have to get out of our self-imposed reality box and just break free. What do you want? If you could *do* anything you wanted or *have* anything you wanted, what would it be? What is the first thing that pops into your mind right now? Don't censor it, don't rationalize it, just allow that thought to come to you. Write it down right here, right now.

If anything were possible, these are my biggest dreams: _____

_____

_____

_____

Let yourself be free enough to dream a bigger dream. I talk to so many people who tell me they don't have really big dreams because they don't know how such big dreams could come true. I am here to tell you the *what* must come before the *how*.

What do you want? It is you placing your "dream order" to God and the universe. It's identifying what you truly want. When you go to a restaurant, what does the waiter ask you? "What can I get for you?" "What would you like to have?" They take your order. They cannot bring you food if you don't place the order. It's the same thing with your dreams. God and the universe cannot deliver what you do not ask for.

Once you know *what* you want, the *how* will start to show up. So many people get this backward. They try to figure out how to get what they want, and when they can't figure out *how* they give up on *what*. I have talked to so many people who have achieved big things in life, and many of them told me that when they started down the path to living their dream, they had no idea how they would make it happen—they just took a step.

If you want to be inspired, read the entire story of how Richard Branson started Virgin Atlantic Airlines. He was stranded in Puerto Rico because his flight to the British Virgin Islands had been canceled. He stated that he wanted to get to the BVI and to the beautiful woman who was waiting there for him. He then began to figure out how. He saw that many people were stranded, so he chartered a plane and wrote on a white board that for thirty-nine dollars you could buy a one-way ticket to the BVI. He filled up the plane, and Virgin Airlines was born.

That is exactly what I did…in a much smaller way. I knew that I wanted to speak and share the message in my heart, but I had no idea *how* that could happen. This was in the early '90s, and we didn't have YouTube or any social media, of course. The only way we had to market was word of mouth and mailing out brochures and videotapes. I knew that if I wanted to be a speaker, the first thing I had to do was write a presentation. So I wrote a presentation. I formed my company, Winners By Choice, I had business cards printed, and I started "acting like" a speaker, even though I had zero speaking gigs on my calendar. I started just letting people know I was available to speak. I started getting calls from different groups asking me what I charged, and I clearly remember saying, "I don't care, whatever you've got." At that point, I truly didn't care about the money. I wasn't chasing the "paper," I was chasing the vision. I believed that I had to just take steps forward.

66 *The WHAT must come before the HOW.* 99

Those steps led me to an event where the owner of a speaker's bureau came to hear me speak and started booking me for a fee. My dedication to the vision was truly leading the way.

Around that same time, after I returned from Mrs. America, I was asked to be a guest on a local morning drive-time radio show in Nashville. It was a very popular morning show, and I was thrilled to be asked to come on for an interview. The interview went so well that the Zoo Crew asked if I would come back each week and do a segment as a guest host. On the spot, I said yes. I had no idea what I would be doing; I just knew I wanted to do it and would figure out how later. I spent several years on the air with Coyote McCloud and The Zoo Crew as the Zoo Mamma. As I write this story, I am reminded that I auditioned to be on the air at my hometown radio station in Eupora to do some reporting on air. It was WEPA, and they didn't hire me. It's clear that dream was alive in my late teens, but I allowed one rejection to stop me. It's just incredible that so many years later I would be on the air in the Nashville prime-time market with a top-rated show. Coyote McCloud is no longer with us, but I smile every time I think of him and the opportunity he gave me. Was I scared at first? Of course I was! I was totally out of my comfort zone. Each week, I had to come up with interesting topics for us to talk about on the air and set up interviews. I learned by doing. I started interviewing some of my favorite authors, and I never knew what would happen on the air doing a live show. I truly believe that experience prepared me for all the things I do now, because I just took the step. I am encouraging you to do the same: just take a step.

Take the First Step

I have continued to learn that important lesson about taking a step forward and facing fear from Nick. I believe it is fear, whether we recognize it or not, that keeps us from attempting to dream and make those dreams come true. Fear throws us all of those questions like, "What if it doesn't work out?" "Why do you believe you are good enough?" "Where will you get the resources, the money, the time, etc.?" Fear paralyzes us from taking the next step.

My unexpected lesson on faith, facing your fear, and taking the next step came on the side of a mountain in Colorado. My entire family was on a ski vacation, and as you have learned earlier in this book, I am not an athletic girl. I am a Southern girl who does not like to be cold! However, on this trip, I was trying to be a good sport and ski with the family because they all love it so much. So I did the right thing—I took a ski lesson and was able to get down the bunny slope without falling. I was pretty proud of myself. Although looking back on that ski lesson, I probably talked more than I skied.

The following day, with all of the voices of encouragement from my family, I decided I could ski one of the green runs with everyone. Trust me, this was such a big deal that my husband skied down the hill to video this adventure. Of course, my son Nick decided to ski down behind me in case there was a tragedy. I was doing great—feeling the wind in my face, feeling so accomplished—when suddenly I ended up in fresh powder; my skis got knocked off my feet and went hurling through the air in one direction, while my body went the other direction. I remember that totally out of control, "Oh Lord, what do I do now?" feeling that happened in a second but felt like hours. I hit the ground, landing flat on my back, and not only did my skis fly, but my glasses flew off my face, my poles went flying, and I was a total hot mess. My husband said later they call it a yard sale, meaning there is just stuff everywhere.

I was lying on the ground, snow in my face, and I swear I could hear the *Wild World of Sports* announcer from years ago in my head saying, "From the thrill of victory to the agony of defeat!" I went from thrill to agony in about two minutes. As I lifted my head from the snow, mascara running down my wet, cold face, I looked around and not only was frustrated but truly scared. All I could see were two-year-olds flying by me without poles, and my feeling of defeat went to an entirely new level. I felt defeated, worthless, and the belief I had held onto for most of my life that I had no athletic ability overtook me. I had broken both of my elbows years earlier from another athletic event. Well, not really; I tripped on my high heels, fell on a sidewalk, and broke them both, but in my head, that was an athletic event. The doctor had told me that if I ever broke them again I would be in surgery. I lay there in the snow that day, paralyzed by fear and frustration, wondering how I would ever get down that mountain in one piece.

All of sudden, I heard skis behind me and snow flying over my head, and I knew it was Nick. In the moments that all of this had happened, I had decided that if I just continued to lie still, the ski patrol would see me, think I was hurt or dead, and get me on a snowmobile. Nick skied up and looked down at me, saying, "Mom, are you OK?"

I looked up and said, "Move on, Nick. I'm waiting for the snowmobile to come rescue me, and if you keep talking to me, the boy won't come." Nick looked down and, in a very strong voice, said, "Mom! Sit up right now." He skied around and gathered all of my stuff. He signaled to my husband that I was OK. He looked down at me again and saw my tears—yes, I said tears. He said, "Mom what is wrong with you?" I shook my head as the mascara-stained tears kept falling. I told him all the fears that had just run through my brain. I was scared of falling and breaking my elbows again; I was scared because I couldn't see the bottom of the mountain. I was scared because I didn't think I could get down the mountain.

Nick skies the double black diamond slopes, so this "yard sale" he found me in seemed ridiculous. He stood there shaking his head at me and quickly said something to me that truly changed my life. He said, "Mom, stop trying to see the bottom of the mountain. Simply ski the two feet in front of you, and when you ski the two feet in front of you, you can ski two more. Before you know it, you will be at the bottom of the mountain, and I will be here to go with you." I honestly wanted to tell him I didn't want his motivational speech on the side of the mountain and this was not a fear I needed to conquer.

But at that moment, I stopped. I remembered all of the life principles I had spent years learning, and in that instant I realized I had an opportunity to learn a new life principle. So I got up, gathered my courage, and did exactly what Nick told me to do. I skied the two feet in front of me, and before I know it we were at the bottom of the mountain. Of course, that video of me on the mountain made for great laughter later and could have ended up on one of those funny video shows.

That boy of mine is very wise. That's how we all have to face our fear and follow our dreams—*ski the two feet in front of us.* You have to take the first step, regardless of how small it is. Our natural reaction to any fear is to step away. My natural reaction to that event was to quit, find a shortcut, and not push myself. I didn't *want* to do it, but I decided to do it anyway. Facing our fear, taking the next step, is not always going to be fun. It's going to be hard, but the only way out of fear is to step into it and move through it. I have thanked Nick many times for forcing me to take a risk and be brave…even when I didn't want to do it.

Do you know the story of J. K. Rowling? If you don't know her name, you do know the name of her books, which have also been made into movies. She is the author of the Harry Potter series. J. K. Rowling went from being a jobless, single mother living off unemployment benefits to one of the best-selling authors of all time. I love her story, because it shows all of us that if we truly follow our dreams, embrace our gifts, and don't give up, anything is possible. She was a divorced mom struggling on welfare who had an idea for a children's book, and she had a dream. She wrote her first and second Harry Potter books from a coffee shop, because it was cheaper to have coffee and write from there than it was to pay her heating bill. She worked hard at her craft before anyone noticed her, because she believed in herself and what she was doing even when it wasn't easy. She faced rejection, but that didn't stop her. After some rejections, she finally sold *Harry Potter and the Sorcerer's Stone* for about $4,000.

By the summer of 2000, the first three books had earned roughly 480 million dollars in three years. As of 2015, the Harry Potter books had been translated into seventy-three different languages, and it was the best-selling book series of all time. The books have also made author J. K. Rowling the highest-paid author in the world. She was the first female to become a billionaire author. I love her story, and I also love this quote from J. K. herself: "Failure meant a stripping away of the inessential. I stopped pretending to myself that I was anything other than what I was and began to direct all my energy into finishing the only work that mattered to me." If you have a dream or passion, don't let rejection and fear stop you. Follow the direction of your heart and don't give up. I hope you will let this story inspire you, and I encourage to read her entire story. It will remind you that anything is possible with a dream, faith, and action!

Vision of Success

Experts have proven that our brains are goal-seeking organisms. Whatever goal, vision, and direction you give your subconscious mind, it will work day and night to achieve it. I am sure you have heard as often as I have about the importance of writing down your goals. We hear that we should do it, but we rarely hear why we should.

Here is the reason that writing down your goals is so important: writing clarifies thought. I remember when I switched from a written day timer to an electronic calendar. All of sudden, I couldn't remember anything. Physically writing something down uses three portions of your brain—visual, motor, and cognitive skills. Did you make notes in school when you were studying for a test? I know I did. I do it now with the books I am reading. I know that if there is an idea I want to remember, writing it down will help me. I have also now come full circle, and I am back to a written calendar and planner, and yes I am remembering what I am writing down.

I have seen statistics that say that only 3 percent of the population writes down their goals. I don't know how scientifically accurate that is, but I do know that as I travel around the world I ask my audiences how many of them have their goals written down on a piece of paper, not in invisible ink in their heads. After the laughter dies down, only about 3 percent of the room raises their hands. I have asked this question in all types of groups—even in sales groups where the participants' careers are based on numbers—and this percentage rarely changes. Why not give yourself the advantage and put in writing what you want for your life? We make grocery lists, we make Christmas lists, we even make lists when we are packing for a trip, so why wouldn't we make a list for our lives? If you have a legally binding document, you always "put it in writing," but so many times we ignore and neglect the biggest deal of all, which is the deal we make with ourselves.

I can't tell you exactly why this works, but I can tell you from personal experience that *it totally works*. I have been "putting it in writing" all of my life. Growing up, I used the written word to write out and process my feelings when I was happy or sad. I have been writing down my goals since my late twenties. I have always embraced the written word. When I was a teenager, we called it a diary, and now as adults, we call it a journal. Now experts everywhere are trying to encourage us to journal, yet so many people push against this simple form of self-expression.

Journaling is an ancient tradition, one that dates back to at least tenth-century Japan. Successful people throughout history have kept journals. Playwright Oscar Wilde said, "I never travel without my diary. One should always have something sensational to read on the train." I love that! There is increasing evidence to support the idea that journaling has a positive impact on physical well-being. For me, through the years I have considered my journals my mental garbage disposal. It's been proven that recalling episodes of anger and frustration with emotion depresses the immune system for up to seven hours. It seems when something frustrating or hurtful happens, people tend to want to process it over and over again. I think it may be for validation that our feelings matter, or perhaps we are hoping for a different outcome.

I have found that if I am having a "character building day," I can write down my frustration and release it from my soul and use that space to start focusing on finding a solution. I may have to write it down more than once to work through it. I have noticed through this process that if I write down exactly what is frustrating me, I can start to find the answers and navigate through it. It's been proven that our brains can only focus on so much at one time. If you are using your mental energy to focus on the things that have happened to you in the past, the problem you are facing, the way someone hurt you, you are robbing yourself of positive, creative energy. Give the answers more focus than the problem.

Scientific evidence proves what I have felt for years. The act of writing accesses your left brain, which is analytical and rational. While your left brain is occupied, your right brain is free to create, intuit, and feel. What does all of that mean? Writing removes mental blocks and allows you to use all of your brainpower to better understand yourself, others, and the world around you. Your journaling is your mental exercise, and it will be most effective if you do it daily for about twenty minutes. Yes, I said twenty minutes. It is my form of prayer, process, and meditation—all rolled into one. I start my days super early with a cup of coffee, my books, and my journal. I can honestly say if my life is super busy and I neglect that "quiet" time, I can totally feel the result in my life. It's as important to my well-being as exercise, sleep, and food.

So many people ask me how to start a journal. Begin anywhere, just start writing and forget spelling and punctuation. Let this be your conversation with yourself, and write anything that you are feeling. However, privacy is key if you are to write uncensored. Write quickly. Why? Because this frees your brain from what you "should" and "shouldn't" write. The most important thing to remember is there is not a right or wrong way to journal.

It fascinated me to learn that many famous people kept journals or diaries. These people came from all walks of life: business (John D. Rockefeller), the military (George Patton), inventors (Benjamin Franklin, Thomas Edison), presidents and prime ministers (John Adams, Ronald Reagan, Winston Churchill), and many authors (Mark Twain, Ernest Hemingway). Eminem keeps a journal. Peyton Manning keeps a journal. Top performers track their progress, set goals, reflect, and learn from their mistakes. I love Julia Cameron's book, *The Artist Way*, in which she guides her readers to write three pages of longhand a day. It's been one of the greatest tools I have ever used in my life. If you want to explore this process, I encourage you to get her book. It's been with me since 1998, and I still refer to it often. Thank you, Julia Cameron, you have truly changed my life.

I am sure you have heard from many different people, including me, about following your dreams, your heart, and your purpose. Those words sound simple, but they are not. Following your heart, your passion and your dreams takes effort. It takes consistent effort, and all of that effort begins in your mind. The longest distance you will ever walk is the eighteen inches from your head to your heart. When your dream goes from just a *head knowledge* to a *heart commitment,* then no one can take it from you or talk you out of it. If it doesn't happen "overnight"—and it usually doesn't—then the heart commitment is what will keep you trying one more time. Jim Carrey had a heart commitment, J. K. Rowling had a heart commitment, and Walt Disney had a heart commitment. What is *your* heart commitment? What dream are you not willing to give up on?

One of the things I have had to learn the hard way is the importance of choosing who you share your dreams with. There are days we are going to doubt ourselves, and on those days, we all need people in our lives who encourage us and believe in us until we can believe in ourselves again. I truly caution you not to share your dreams with people who are not dreamers themselves. Why? Because they will not understand. I want you to protect your dream just like you would protect a newborn baby. This is your newborn dream, and exposing it to people who are not dreamers and believers is like exposing a newborn to people with the flu. You would never bring a newborn into a room of very sick people, yet many people expose their newborn dreams to people who are carrying the dream-killing disease of doubt. Who is the *one* person in your life that you can share your dream with?

My Dream Keeper is: _____ .

Write that person's name down and let them know that he or she is your *Dream Keeper.* If you don't have anyone in your world, then *I will be your dream keeper.* I want you to feel free to email me your dream at Dale@winnersbychoice.com.

You may find it hard to believe, but even with all of the work and teaching that I do, there are times I am faced with doubt and uncertainty about my dreams. It was hard for me to turn over this manuscript. My manager finally forced me to give it to him to read. He said, "Send me your manuscript." There was no discussion. He simply told me to send it. He is the person representing me, my brand, and my message. I knew he had to read it, but I couldn't believe the panic I was feeling knowing that someone else would have my dream in their hands. But because I trust him and know he has my best interests at heart, I could let it go and know that anything he said to me would come from a place of support, not criticism. That is exactly what happened with the edits with the book. Both Ross and my amazing editor, Susan, gently guided me back to my voice when I strayed from it. It was never easy to send it to either of them, and I faced fear each time. But there are times you just have to follow the instructions of Nike and "Just Do It."

If you doubt yourself or your dreams and you don't have someone to believe in you, pour positive inspiration into your soul and read stories of people who have overcome the odds to make their dreams a reality. Read the story of Michael Jordan and how his tenth-grade coach cut him from the team and told him he was too small to play. Read the story of Rocky himself, Sylvester Stallone. He was broke, homeless, and even had to sell his dog for twenty-five dollars to buy food. He was inspired by watching a boxing match between Mohammad Ali and Chuck Wepner. It took him twenty hours to write the first *Rocky* script. He not only wanted to sell the script, but he wanted to star in the movie. However, each studio kept telling him that they wanted his script but they wanted a "real" star to play Rocky. He refused, and eventually they agreed to allow him to star in the movie—and the rest is history. Sly was committed in his heart to his passion. Now, all these years later, he recently received his first Golden Globe award for the movie *Creed* at age sixty-nine.

These are just a few of the many, many stories of people who have overcome the odds to follow their dreams. The question is, "Are you willing to do whatever it takes to follow your personal dreams?" What is your dream I.Q.? Dream I.Q. is your *I Quit* resolve. Are you willing to make this statement: I will, *until!* You will fight for your dream *until* you see it come to pass, or you will fight for your dream *until* you change the direction of your dream. You may start out following a dream, and as you grow and change you are led to something more.

My Dream I.Q. is: _____ .

As I close this chapter, I want you to ask yourself if you have given yourself the permission to dream…*really* dream? If not, I hope today as you read this book that this will be the spark that ignites something within your soul. If your dream is to write a book, I believe there is someone out there who is supposed to read that book. If you sing or act or speak, then I believe there is someone out there who is supposed to hear from you. If you write movies, or design video games, or build buildings, someone is waiting for you. Don't rob the world of the gift you are meant to share. Get started now!

If you aren't sure what your real dreams are, I suggest that you simply get curious. Pay attention to what fascinates you. Stop and pay attention to things you enjoy that catch your attention. As I said, Nick had his car fascination from a very young age, and I was always fascinated with actors, actresses, and people who were on stage. I didn't give those thoughts any power in my pursuit of a college degree, because I discredited those dreams before I ever gave them a chance. Start your dream-building process today. It doesn't matter how old you are, where you live, or what you do for a living right now. Dream-building is free, and it is fun. If you want to be a writer, sit down with an author and ask some questions. If you want to be an actress, take a class. My gorgeous friend Rebecca is such an inspiration to me. After raising her children and going through a divorce at age fifty, she started following her dream of being an actress. I am happy to say that Rebecca is living her dream now, in television and film, and every time I see her on Facebook, she is in another movie. I just love it.

Dreams, goals, and visions can only come true if you decide to face your fear, whatever it may be. It requires being a risk taker. It requires stepping out of your comfort zone, and that is not always easy. I challenge you, really challenge you, whatever dream you are pursuing, whatever fear you are facing, to remember the words of Nick Thomas: "Ski the two feet in front of you." Each step you take will encourage you and empower you to take the next step. This is your life; these are your dreams. Make them a reality, Gorgeous!

66 The only place your dream becomes impossible is in your own thinking. 99

ROBERT SCHULLER

66 All things splendid have been achieved by those who dared believe that something inside them was superior to circumstance. 99

BRUCE BARTON

66 It had long since come to my attention that people of accomplishment rarely sat back and let things happen to them. They went out and happened to things. 99

LEONARDO DA VINCI

137

Take Aways

_____

_____

_____

_____

_____

_____

_____

_____

_____

_____

_____

_____

_____

_____

_____

_____

_____

Take Aways

Empower yourself and others to find the light from within and let it shine.

GIFT SIX

Turn on the Light

#GMG

Light, Listen, Learn

You may be wondering what in the world those three words have to do with each other. In addition to the other life principles I have shared with you, these three words are the three concepts that have made a difference for me. In the darkest times of my life, when I felt lost and didn't feel gorgeous inside or out, I had to find a way to stand in the light of truth. I had to listen to those I trusted to help me when I felt lost and unsure, and more importantly, I had to listen to myself. I had to learn to trust myself and learn to honor the gifts God has given me and the dreams that have been placed in my heart.

Why is light so important? I believe light is important because when we truly embrace the light, darkness must disappear. Darkness cannot drive out darkness—only light can do that. Darkness is not an opponent for the light. It must always disappear. Even a little light starts to change darkness.

I will share with you in the final chapter some of the darkest, most confusing times of my life. When you face unexpected situations that bring confusion and uncertainty, and your life feels overcast and dark, it is hard not to simply go with that darkness, to the think the worst. When the darkness of our mind starts to creep in, we begin to imagine things and think things that are not true. Remember when you were a little kid and you imagined so many things in the dark. You constantly saw things that weren't there. That is what happens when we embrace the darkness; it distorts our thinking, and we believe things that are not true. We begin to think of the worst possible scenario, and our mind and body start to react to that. We begin to worry about things that aren't real—that may not happen—but we distress ourselves with the possibility.

If you have experienced this, you are not alone. Even five hundred years ago, Michel de Montaigne said, "My life has been filled with terrible misfortune; most of which never happened." Science has now proven that 85 percent of what we worry about never happens and the 15 percent that does happen, most people find they can handle it much better than expected…or it teaches them a valuable lesson. What that tells us is that 97 percent of what we are worrying about is created by our fearful mind, which exaggerates our circumstances and our ability to handle it.

Fortunately for me, when I was facing a physical and emotional crisis, I had been doing the personal development work for years, and I knew that my thoughts and fears could not be trusted. I knew that the biggest battle was between my ears—in my mind. I knew that if I gave those thoughts power they would grow and get stronger. If I fed them with the fuel of attention, they would get stronger and more powerful. Each and every time my negative thoughts and the darkness wanted to consume me with the worst possible outcome, I stood up inside myself, searched for the light of truth, and gave it my focus.

When we feel broken and damaged, it is so easy to let the diminishing thoughts of darkness rule. When we are afraid and unsure of ourselves and our future, it's so easy to let the darkness take over. It takes a *decision* to fight for the light. It takes discipline to stay strong when you feel like crumbling. It takes a daily decision to fight for the truth. What is the light of truth? The truth is if you are still blessed to be breathing and wake up to see the light of day, *anything* is possible. The truth is if you are reading these words and holding this book, anything is possible. The truth is you were created to live the dreams that have been ignited in your soul.

Think about plants. They don't grow in darkness; they need light. Darkness is doubt. Your soul can't grow in darkness. Your faith, your potential, or your possibilities can't grow in darkness. None of them can grow in darkness. What grows in darkness then? Fear grows in darkness; confusion, doubt, and feeling powerless grows in darkness. I once read that there is no visibility at point blank range. What does that mean? It means if you are only focused on the darkness, you can't see past that darkness. What you focus on truly gets bigger. When you find one reason that something will stop you, you can find five more. But, it also works the other way. If you can find one truth about yourself, about your situation, about your possibilities, then you can find one more. As we explored in an earlier chapter, the words you are using to talk to yourself either make the days darker or they help the light to ascend.

The thoughts and beliefs that will change your life need light. The thoughts and life principles that can and will change your life need to be nourished and fed daily. There will be times in your life that the only thing you may have is faith. There were days during some of my toughest challenges that I wasn't sure how I'd make it. But each day, I got up and found the light of faith. Each day, I found one possibility, and not only did I make it—my life has flourished since that time. I made a choice to find the light in the middle of heartache, confusion, and uncertainty. I made a choice to find the light, and you can too, whatever you are facing right now, whatever challenge is in your life. I am lovingly guiding you to find the light. Every day we choose our destiny. Every day we get to make choices. I had to make small choices every day to find my self-worth again, to rediscover myself. I did it; no, it wasn't always easy, but it was worth it.

When we are broken, we usually ask two questions: "Why is this happening to me?" and "How could this happen to me?" Those thoughts, those questions keep us bound to the past, and they keep us asking questions that have no answers. The only question that can bring answers into your life is this one: "What can I do right now to bring more light, joy, hope, faith, happiness, gratitude, and peace into my life?" What can I do right now to move forward, even if it is just my attitude and outlook? There will be times in all of our lives when the *only* thing we can change is our attitude and our outlook. We can't control other people, we can't control many circumstances, but we can control our reaction to those things. Do not appraise a situation in your life based on your memory of the past or your fear of the future. Make a *right now* decision. I am not talking about setting goals or anything like that. I am just talking about getting yourself to the next moment when you are facing a difficult time.

Notice I didn't say ask yourself what you can do *tomorrow, next week, or next year.* When we walk through difficult times, we have to know and understand that we may not even see the possibility of change coming in our lives, so the point of power is in the present moment. You can turn more light on in your life by reading something that inspires you for ten minutes. You can turn more light on in your life with gratitude. Gratitude will instantly take you from darkness to light. You can turn more light on in your life by talking to someone who truly supports you and encourages you. (REVISIT your list of what you are grateful for.) It's that simple and that hard. It is simple because they are easy things to do, and it's hard because when we are in the middle of a dark situation, we have to *remember* to make a choice to find something positive.

For me, when I have faced the most difficult times, I just wanted to hide and turn inward. Even though I knew that was not what would help me, it was my natural instinct. I had to make myself seek out what I knew would help me improve, even when I didn't want to or didn't feel like it. There were times I didn't feel like looking for something positive in the midst of the struggle. When your energy is drained, and you feel depleted, it takes real discipline to make that step.

Once a glass, a vase, or any object has been broken, it never goes back to its exact original state. You may be able to put it back together well enough that no one ever knows it's been broken, but it is not the same. If you have been through an experience that hurt you and you felt broken from it, you can't expect to be exactly as you were before that experience. It's not possible. But you have two choices in any experience that robs you of your joy and hurts your soul—you can let it defeat you (darkness) or define you (light).

Even when the experience has been heartbreaking, hard, and difficult, if you can learn from the experience, grow from it, then I urge you step into gratitude. I have said over and over for years that for each experience we face, we can either just *go* through it or *grow* through it. The pain you walked through was just the tuition you paid for your great life lesson. You may feel like I've felt at times; I've wanted to say, "Hey, life, that was not the way I wanted to learn that lesson." Unfortunately, we don't get to choose how most of our life lessons show up for us.

One of the things I did through the years when I was feeling defeated and confused was to have a strong talk with myself, just like I would with a friend who I loved. I hope you will take these words and write them down. I would write them in my journal over and over again, and I would read them out loud. I would keep planting the seed of truth in my soul. Let this be your light in the darkness. Speak the truth to your soul, and even though I don't know you personally, I *know* these words are truth—and they can be your light. Write them down. Repeat them out loud. Let them sink into your soul.

I will not allow any relationship or situation to be the reflection of my self-worth. I am a woman of enormous substance and faith. I am a woman of compassion, intelligence, vision, beauty, influence, strength, generosity, and soul. My future and my happiness are determined by these things—who I am, what I think, and what I choose. Right now, at this moment, I respect myself, I honor myself, and I choose to be the best possible version of myself. I choose light in the middle of darkness. I choose faith in the middle of fear. I choose belief in the middle of doubt. I choose clarity in the middle of confusion. I choose to be a victor and not a victim. I choose to honor my gorgeous spirit inside and out. I choose myself.

> *I will NOT allow any relationship or situation to be the reflection of my self-worth.*

Those words may not feel like your truth right now, and they will never be if you don't start to embrace them. It took me so long to realize that choosing myself was not selfish—it was required if I wanted to continue to give to others. I had to stop and ask myself what I was feeling and what I needed. I'm still not good at that, but I continue to work on it daily. Regardless of how it feels, speak these words to your soul, and speak them over and over again until you truly start to believe them. The action is the cure for changing what you feel.

Listen with Your Heart

If you are a parent, I am sure you have asked this question as many times as I have over the years: "Are you listening to me?" We have told our kids over and over and over again to listen to us. We want them to hear what we are telling them. I want to ask you the same question: *Are you listening?* You may be confused by that question, and you may be saying right back to me, *Listening to what?* Well, are you listening to the most important person in your life: yourself? In this great adventure in life, we are told what to do from childhood, and then we continue to seek the opinions and thoughts of others throughout our lives. Along the way, especially in times of confusion and uncertainty, it's so hard to trust ourselves and listen to ourselves. It's hard to trust our intuition.

Sometimes, when I am faced with difficult situations, I just want someone to tell me what to do. There have been times in my life I've been so exhausted from trying to "figure it out" that I just wanted someone to make it easy for me. Unfortunately, easy is not an option. When you are moving forward in your life, making big life decisions, changing your life, and pushing out of your comfort zone, no one can tell you what to do. I totally believe in getting counsel from people you trust when you need advice. I have a small group of people I turn to if I am challenged with a decision, but at the end of the day, regardless of what they tell me, it is my inner guidance that I must trust.

Guidance and advice are not the same. Your guidance, your truth, your real answers must come from within. The advice comes from outside of you from other sources. Guidance is an inside job. Before you quickly take the advice of someone else about your life, stop, pause, and seek your guidance to see if that suggestion rings true for you. I don't believe that guidance can be heard in the midst of noise and chaos. If you want to be led and you want to hear, you have to get quiet—and that means by yourself. It doesn't mean with the television or music in the background, notifications going off on your phone, or kids screaming in the background. It means giving yourself the gift of quiet. I read recently that both *listen* and *silent* use the same letters. There is a lot of power in that statement. You can't listen to someone else talk to you if you are not silent, and you can't hear your soul speaking to you if you aren't allowing yourself the gift of silence.

I think many times we pray for answers, but we do not stop and give ourselves the space to listen to them. Meditation has gotten to be a huge thing in our culture. More people are turning to yoga and meditation than ever before. I will have to admit that I did not understand meditation or the power of it until the past few years. I remember when I first started trying this practice, I truly thought it couldn't possibly be hard. I figured I could sit still for ten minutes, focus on my breathing, and just let my brain be still. Wow, was I wrong. Suddenly, after just a few minutes, I realized that even though I was sitting there quietly, my brain was two days ahead in the next speaking engagement or two days behind in a conversation that had left me unsettled. I noticed quickly where I was not; I was *not* present. I was way ahead or way behind, and it has taken practice to be able to quiet my mind. Meditation is simply awareness. Our minds and our lives are on overload, and that overload creates stress that is leading to illness. We have so many thoughts running through our minds, and most of them we aren't even aware of. Whatever you do with awareness is meditation. I think it is simply taking the time to step out of the chaos of life and be "totally aware" in the present moment. When I sit quietly and journal, I consider that part of my meditation. I think meditation is as individual as the people who choose to embrace it. I feel like it's the path to shutting out the noise in our mind so we can hear our soul.

Like anything else, meditation takes practice. Sitting quietly for two minutes without letting your brain just run from thought to thought is a skill. But the benefits are huge. Science is now proving that if we make a habit of quieting our minds in some way, it relieves our stress, and stress is the main contributor to chronic illness. But how many people will say, "I don't have time to sit quietly for ten minutes," even though they have time for the evening news, checking Facebook, or watching their favorite television show? No, it's not about time, it is about choice. I love this old zen saying, "You should sit every day for twenty minutes unless you're too busy. Then you should sit for an hour." What I have learned to do that works for me is to pause and be aware. I can be sitting on a plane waiting for takeoff, and I can close my eyes, just focus on my breathing, and let go of the to-do list in my brain for a few moments. I don't have to be in my house or sitting on the floor. I can do that if I have time, but "geography" is not going to be my excuse not to turn to the quiet.

I truly believe that if you start with two minutes a day, make that a habit, and then move to ten minutes a day, you will learn to open up that quiet space; and in that quiet space, you can begin to listen more to your inner guidance. Go into that quiet space with the situations that you need to receive guidance for and then listen. I always jot down what I feel like I am being led to do during that quiet time. I love the scripture passage "Be still and know that I am God." I think to see anything clearly we have to find that stillness. Think about the mirror on your wall. Could you sit in front of it and do your makeup or hair with the mirror moving? Of course you couldn't. You can't see your reflection in the waves of the ocean, but you can see your reflection in a pool of still water. Stillness brings things into focus. Stillness in your soul will help bring your life into focus. Stillness will help bring you the answers you need for your life.

I have shared about light and listening, and now it's time for the big *L:* learning. I know many people think that the learning ends when you graduate, get the diploma, and launch into life. For me, that was just the beginning. My college degree was an accomplishment, but only because I had completed college. The physical education degree is such a beacon to me that I had no clue of who I was or what I wanted to do with my life. It's OK that I didn't know what I wanted to do, but the wider choice was that I chose to go against every instinct and personal gift that I had. I did not listen and learn at that time of my life. In my heart, I knew it didn't feel right. I knew it wasn't my heart's desire. I knew it wasn't my skill set. It is still laugh out loud funny to me that I have a degree in physical education when I have zero, and I mean zero, athletic ability. I can't dribble a basketball; I can't hit a volleyball over a net; and watching me swing a golf club should be on some video blooper television show. It's *not* my gift.

I understand and love sports, but I am not the girl you'd pick for your intramural team. But through the years I've had to learn the lessons that all of my life experiences have brought me. I mentioned the lesson my son Nick taught me on the side of the ski mountain, but he taught me another lesson at the top of a rappelling tower in the jungle in Mexico. During a family vacation, we had decided to do an adventure day that was to include snorkeling, cave swimming, rappelling, and zip-lining. I had secretly told myself I'd be a good sport and do the swimming part but would bail on the jungle rappelling and zip-lining adventure. I made it through the two swimming experiences, but not without a near interaction with a barracuda.

When it was time to climb the seventy-foot tower that we would be rappelling down, both of my bonus children (my husband's children) decided it was not for them. They are not comfortable with heights, and rappelling off that tower was not anything they wanted to do. They declined and told the rest of our group to have fun. They were in their twenties at the time, and I thought Nick would give me a hall pass on this since they didn't feel comfortable going. No, of course he didn't. He totally challenged me to try it, and once again I had no good reason to tell him I wouldn't do it. It was one of those special mother/son moments that I knew needed to happen. I also knew it was a learning moment for me. Could I put into practice all of these life principles that I teach around the world on a rappelling tower in a Mexican jungle?

As we climbed this tower, I was trying to keep my mind calm. My mind would start to drift to the reality of this experience, and I could feel the panic start to rise. Each time it did, I had to do exactly what I have written about in this book. I had to take control of my thoughts and choose not to think about the reality of hanging seventy feet in the air on the side of a tower. If you are a sports person, and especially if you are an extreme sports person, I'm sure it seems ridiculous that I would be so unnerved by this, but this is totally out of my comfort zone. I have told people over and over that my version of climbing new heights is to wear the five-inch heels instead of the four.

When you are about to face a big challenge, you have to stay 100 percent present on whatever you are doing at that present moment. My focus as I climbed that tower was honestly one step at a time. I forced myself not to even glance down and see how high we were. I knew if I did it, it would be over. I knew if I allowed myself that one glance, my fear and doubt would get the attention they were screaming for and I would be walking back down that tower. Again, all the life lessons I had learned kicked in, and I focused on the fact that I knew that Nick would not put me in danger. I focused on the fact that people did this every day many times a day, and they were fine. I focused on the fact that in the scope of life challenges, this was small stuff. I was the one making it big stuff!

As we neared the top, I saw the other people who were going before me, and I saw what was really about to happen. I was going to be harnessed in, but to rappel down the tower, the first step I was going to take out of that tower was backward. I truly froze. Somewhere in observation of this activity, I had failed to recognize that you had to step out backward to go down backward. Nick immediately saw the look on my face and said this, "Mom, look at me. Just look at me, and do exactly what I tell you to do. You can do this." As he helped me into the harness, he kept repeating that to me. "Mom, don't look down, don't look around, just look at me, and I will tell you exactly what to do. Trust me." In the middle of my fear, it was my moment to totally trust my son. I did exactly as he told me and stepped off the seventy-foot tower backward, never letting my eyes leave his eyes. I had to put my faith in him when I had zero faith in myself. If he believed I could do it, then I could do it. I did do it. I doubt you'll ever see me there again, but I did it.

There were several lessons in that experience, with the most prominent one being if you are petrified by fear, don't get too far ahead of yourself and start trying to predict the future. I could not even allow myself to look around. I had to focus on putting one foot in front of me as I climbed higher and higher. I knew the moment I looked down and took the first sip of doubt that it would be poison to my confidence and my belief. Once I got to the top, I had to trust Nick. I knew he loved me, and he had done it so many times before. I had to once again look at him, look at the belief in his eyes, and trust that belief. I never did look down as I stepped off that tower.

When you are in the middle of doubt, in the middle of a crisis, if you can find that one person who believes in you and lock into his or her belief until you have built back your own, it will change you. If you can, find one person who will listen and really *hear* you. I think many people can have conversations, but truly hearing someone requires not just your ears but your heart. In so many different experiences in my life, it's been one person's belief that turned me back around when I was experiencing self-doubt. So I have learned that when I am gripped with fear, doubt, hesitation, and uncertainty, instead of running from that experience, I need to take one step forward and find at least one person who will believe for me and with me as I move forward.

Each difficulty in your life holds a lesson for you. The most difficult times in my life have brought the most powerful lessons. At times, I saw the lesson instantly and navigated much more quickly. At other times in my life, it's been years later—after being willing to learn more about myself and ask the tough questions—that I have learned the lesson.

I do believe that life will continue to present to you experiences that are meant to teach you the lesson you need for your life until you learn it. Pay attention. Be a good student of life. Don't be lazy in learning. Life doesn't have to beat you down for you to learn. You can learn through joy, but it seems it is pain that gets our attention much faster.

I challenge you to do what I have done along the way. Look at each situation and think about what the lesson was at that moment and how you can use that lesson to move your life forward or how you can help someone else. List those experiences here and the lesson learned. Look at the painful events in your life, and identify that one takeaway that can teach you. Look at the joyful times in your life and what that lesson also taught you.

These experiences taught me these lessons:

_____

_____

_____

_____

_____

_____

_____

_____

The other component of learning is learning from others. It is one of the reasons I read as much as I do. I read to learn from others. I know that many people who have gone before me have had experiences that can teach me—as long as I am willing to listen and learn. We are influenced and affected by the people we surround ourselves with throughout our lives. It is so true that those who do not increase us will decrease us. Get tough with yourself and ask yourself if the people you spend the most time with are builders or destroyers. Builders talk about ideas, encouragement, and inspiration, and destroyers talk about other people.

I have to admit that one of my best qualities is believing in the potential in others. However, that belief system has also led me to remain in relationships, both personal and professional, that were not in my best interest and that were not a positive influence in my life. But I had to learn the lesson and see it for myself. There may be relationships in your life that you need to bless with love, release, and let go. If you have a friend who is negative and for whom everything is gloom and doom, you can still love that person, but you need to limit your time with her. If you have a coworker who is constantly complaining, don't be the space where he can just dump all of the negativity. Let others know that you will let them "identify" the problem (which can usually be done in five minutes or less), but you want to empower solutions. If you are solution focused, the people who just want to complain will begin to understand very quickly that you are not the person they can come to and just complain. They will stop doing it once you have set the boundary.

You get to choose the "input" that you listen to. Become aware of the people in your world and ask yourself if you are learning from them, being encouraged by them, and being understood by them. Are they draining you with their energy or building you up with their energy? Learn what empowers you and what drains you, and make a choice to surround yourself with life-building forces.

This section is about learning, and I want to personally mention some of the teachers in my life that I have learned from through the years. I challenge you to research these authors. They are light givers. I want to personally say thank you to Zig Ziglar, Denis Waitley, Les Brown, Tony Robbins, Nido Qubein, Larry Winget, Og Mandino, Napoleon Hill, Jack Canfield, Mark Victor Hanson, and Jeff Olson. Thank you also to Oprah Winfrey, Barbara DeAngelis, Sarah Ban Breathnach, Elizabeth Gilbert, Louise Hay, Marianne Williamson, Gabbie Bernstein, Julia Cameron, Danielle Laporte, and Christiane Northrup.

Be There

I love looking at the names of all of these authors, and these are just a few of the many I have learned from in the past twenty-five years. I love Napoleon Hill's book *Think and Grow Rich,* written in 1937. One of my favorite concepts he wrote about was creating a mastermind alliance. In *The Master-Key to Riches,* Napoleon Hill says, "Every mind needs friendly contact with other minds, for food of expansion and growth." If you have someone in your life who will truly connect with you and share ideas with you about your dreams and goals, don't take that for granted. Spend time together creating a mastermind partnership and helping each other. If you find someone who truly "gets you" and understands your goals and dreams, and you can understand theirs, it creates a special kind of synergy that can't be explained. It truly can take your life to an entirely different level. Many successful people refer to this principle, and I urge you to learn more about it.

But what if you don't have that and can't find it? What if you have those people in your world, but time prohibits you from having those conversations on a regular basis? Honestly, that is what has happened to me through the years. I am blessed with some true mastermind partnerships, but due to all of our schedules, it's always hard to find the time to step out of the demands of life and give that attention to each other.

I realized recently that those relationships I value so much are the same qualities I need to have with myself and with my dream. Whether I get to have conversations with others or not, I need to show up for myself and for the calling that I know I have been put on this earth to fulfill.

How do you do that? How do you show up for yourself and your dream? First of all, you treat it with the same respect that you do the relationships that you value. What do you do for the people that you value? You make time for them. You take the time to listen and engage. You give your attention.

We have to do that for ourselves. When is the last time you gave *yourself* the attention that you give to those you care about and love? I know it's hard for me. I always feel like I should be doing something for someone else. What about your dreams, your passion, and your life? Treat those dreams and that calling like you would treat someone you love.

For me, it means that I have to give my writing, working on my presentations, and building my product line the same kind of attention that I give my closest inner circle. It means that I honor those dreams by giving them the time they need and deserve to grow.

Because I love the interaction and integrated conversation, and I love creating with someone else, it is not always easy being a solo entrepreneur. But if you truly have a dream and passion, you are not alone. You are on the path of creation with the dream you have been given, and it deserves your time and attention. Honor it. You honor it by setting time aside just for it.

If you are a writer, set aside time to write, even if it is for fifteen minutes. Show up for that talent and that dream. If you are a singer, set aside time to sing, even if it's just for yourself. Show your dream that you are *all in,* and show your dream that you respect it and honor it and will not neglect it.

How do relationships die? Neglect. How do plants die? Neglect. How does your health deteriorate? Neglect. Everything in your life is either growing or dying. Everything in your life is either in expansion or contraction. Your dreams and the power of them will contract if you do not give them the attention they need. Relationships can't survive if you only give them attention now and then. Great relationships, talent, and dreams are built by giving them attention on a consistent basis.

Don't let the habit of neglect rob you of the dreams and talents you were sent to this planet to share. Nurture, build, protect, and defend those dreams. Treat them like the most important relationships in your life, because they are. They will never leave you. This is truly the *one* relationship that you are in total control of. You don't have to wait for your dreams to show up and be present. They are *always* waiting on you. You are their protector and their defender. You decide if they grow and flourish or if they die. You have all the power over those dreams.

What will you choose?

Some women are lost in the fire; some women are built from it. There is no darkness so dense, so menacing, or so difficult that it cannot be overcome by light.

VERN P. STANFILL

People are like stained-glass windows. They sparkle and shine when the sun is out, but when the darkness sets in, their true beauty is revealed only if there is light from within.

ELISABETH KÜBLER-ROSS

Take Aways

_____

_____

_____

_____

_____

_____

_____

_____

_____

_____

_____

_____

_____

_____

_____

_____

Take Aways

"*Always wear your invisible crown.***"**

LILLY PULITZER

GIFT SEVEN

Chin Up, Crown Up

#GMG

Where's Your Crown?

As we come to the end of this book and our time together, I have a question for you: "Where's your crown?" I know that may seem like a ridiculous question. You may be saying immediately, "Come on, Dale. I don't have a crown." You may not have a physical crown, but I want to show and guide you to the fact that you do have an invisible crown. I know that I wasn't aware of mine for a very long time. I can certainly tell you where my old rhinestone crown is that once was on my head during the year I was Mrs. Tennessee. It's sitting on the shelf in my bookcase in my office. It's missing rhinestones, and it's so bent that I'm not sure it could sit on anyone's head anymore. Why is it missing rhinestones, and why is it bent? Because during my year as Mrs. Tennessee, I took it off over and over again to let little girls who were fascinated with it put it on their heads. I am not sure we girls ever lose our fascination with sparkly things.

The year I was Mrs. Tennessee, Nick was four, and I took him with me to almost every public appearance. I took him to the parades, the fairs, and the autograph signings. In fact, Nick was signing autographs himself at age four. I remember one particular day like it was yesterday. Nick was with me while I was making an appearance at the Peach Festival in West Tennessee. Suddenly, in the middle of the event, he had to go to the bathroom, and it had to be at that moment. I grabbed his sweet little hand and, in high heels with a crown on my head, off to the bathroom we went. Of course, I was in a hurry to get back to the table where I was greeting everyone, so I didn't even think when I bent over to help him pull up his pants. You can guess what happened next—that crown fell off my head and went right in the toilet.

I will never forget Nick's laughter that day. This adorable, fat little four-year-old giggling, pointing, and saying, "Mommy your crown is in the potty." What do you do? You fish it out, wash it off, and put it back on your head. I didn't realize it at the time, but there was a huge life lesson at that moment. The invisible crowns that we all wear occasionally get knocked off and fall in the toilet or get kicked across the floor. What we then do is we have to dig deep within and find a way to pick them up and put them back on our heads. We have to find a way to do it for ourselves. We can't wait for someone to do that for us.

I love acronyms. I have them for everything. I started thinking about the definition of a crown and what it means. Here is my definition of CROWN:

Confidently

Respecting

Our

Worth

NOW!

How do you know when your crown is slipping and you are not respecting your self-worth? You pay attention to how it feels. It is simple. If you feel confident, strong, powerful in a positive way, kind, loving, and joyful, you are respecting yourself, and your crown is on your head and shining brightly. If you are feeling defeated, unsure, manipulated, sad, and unworthy, look within— your crown has slipped. When you do not confidently respect your worth right now, the crown slides off; at times, it's hard to get it back on your head.

I believe we all come to this planet with that invisible crown on our heads. I believe those personal crowns are a gift from God, and they are custom made. Your crown is only for you. It will *never* fit anyone else. It's *your* special crown. That crown represents all of your uniqueness, your talents, and your gifts. Think about this, how do you keep a crown on your head? You have to hold your head up. To hold your head up, you have to feel confident that God not only gave you that crown, but He also gave you all the personal, unique, and special traits that go with your crown. These invisible crowns are not made of rhinestones—they are made with discipline, determination, faith, self-confidence, self-worth, and a huge amount of courage. The courage to know yourself, love yourself, and realize that you are the queen of your life. You have the choice to live your life to the fullest.

> 66 *Wear your crown proudly as it represents all of your uniqueness, talents, and gifts.* 99

Many children, especially those under the age of four, walk around with their heads held high, totally confident in who they are. They sing out loud; they dance, they play, they tell us their biggest dreams. They don't stop to wonder if anyone likes their singing or their dreams or approves of them—all that matters is whether it feels good to them. The crown may be bouncing around on their pretty little heads, but it hasn't fallen off, because they haven't dipped their heads in self-doubt yet. They don't care if their singing is off-key or if they are dancing in a silly way. They are simply embracing what feels right in their soul. They have never considered doubting who they truly are. They have never disrespected their opinion of themselves.

What does that mean? How do we disrespect ourselves? The moment someone else's opinion of us starts to matter more than our own, we bow our heads in disrespect to who we are and our crowns fall off. We listen to what someone says about how we look, or our talent, or any opinion they have of us, and we start to doubt ourselves. We give more credit to their viewpoint than our own.

As we get older, we may start to wonder "what are they thinking," and those voices can become the loudest voices in our lives. I think many times when we are sure someone is thinking about us, they are not thinking about us at all. They are thinking about their own problems and issues. When we give our attention to what someone else "could be" thinking, then we have taken our eyes off being the best version of ourselves. We have to understand and accept that we are never going to please everyone. It's going to be a lifelong journey that we will have to make to check in with ourselves and find out what *we* think and make our decisions based on that!

Many times, I have allowed someone to disrespect me, we all have. What I had to understand about that was when I allowed that person to disrespect me, I disrespected myself. Disrespecting myself caused my soul to shut down, and I turned inward. I didn't speak up for myself, I started questioning myself, and I began to doubt myself. I allowed that opinion to be my reality. The key word is *allowed*. No one can make you feel angry, disappointed, sad, or defeated without your consent. The biggest lesson about those times in my life for me was that, like most of us, I wasn't even aware that it was happening; I just knew it did not feel good in my soul.

I have had extremely painful moments in my life that honestly changed me. During those times, I didn't understand fully that it would be those extreme moments of pain that would make me stronger and kinder and show me the strength I possessed. At those moments when I felt defeated, I had to dig deep to find my faith. There were times I felt defeated over things that were big life experiences and times I felt defeated over things that just hurt my feelings.

At those times, I had to remember that God would see me through if I would pay attention. I had to remember that the light would win.

Each experience you and I walk through can either defeat us or define us. Queens know that pain is inevitable in life, but suffering is optional. Each experience you face presents a choice to *go* through it or *grow* through it. Each time you grow, your crown stays on your head and you become stronger. Each time your crown stays on your head, you learn to trust yourself. When you trust yourself, you follow your dreams and goals and live your life's purpose. We are not going to go through life without pain or discomfort, so it is our choice to let it teach us, not terrify us.

> 66 *You have the choice to live*
> *your life to the fullest.* 99

If you are a woman who walks in absolute confidence every day of your life, I honor you. But if you are like the rest of us who struggle, you just need to understand that this journey to self-esteem, self-worth, and self-respect is a never-ending journey. There will always be some event, some person with the power to knock your crown off your head onto the floor and kick it across the room. However, when that crown starts to slip, it's your responsibility to recognize it, put your hand to your head, and straighten it.

How do you straighten your crown? First, you recognize that it's in jeopardy of coming off, that you are standing at the crossroads of choice: to choose your self-esteem and respect or not. All of this happens in a nanosecond, and usually the default program we run in our brain is the one that supports the crown falling off. The default program is almost always our negative programming.

Why is the negative programming the default program? It is because it's the one that gets the most use. It's the automatic "go-to." The language goes like this, "Of course he didn't call you back, why would he?" "It *always* happens to you." "Of course you didn't get that job, why would they hire you?" "Look at you. You are not pretty enough, smart enough . . ." Once that assault starts with the negative dialogue, you must be disciplined enough to stop that thought process.

We are all going to go through difficult times; pain will cause us to pay attention to the moment, and it will teach us if we are willing to learn. It's taken years and years for me to understand what it "feels like" and what it does to my soul and my body when I bow my head and my crown falls off. We have to pay attention to how it feels in our soul. Each time I have doubted myself and bowed my head in defeat, my crown has fallen off. Each time I have not stood up for myself, I bowed my head and my crown fell off. Each time I didn't protect my personal boundaries, I bowed my head and my crown fell off. And now I recognize that, without exception, if I allow myself to go down that path of personal disrespect, I get a migraine. My body will instantly show me what is going on and get my attention.

No one can disrespect you, make you mad, make you feel guilty, take your dreams, or destroy your self-worth and self-esteem without your consent. When you bow your head and accept their truth, your crown tumbles to the floor.

When you start to feel invisible, defeated, and unattractive and you feel that you are not valuable, *stop* and pay attention to your language and your actions. What have you allowed that has caused this reaction in your soul? Your soul is mourning the fact that you have walked away from the queen that you are. It is true that we will all turn away from who we are from time to time, but the bigger question is, How long will you allow yourself to stay there? It is up to us to reach for the highest within ourselves, and when we reach for the highest in ourselves, then we empower others by our actions to reach for their highest calling. When we step away from who we are, it doesn't just affect us, it affects those around us.

> **❝** *Queens are never victims—they are victors.* **❞**

One of the most powerful turning points in my life came just a few years after winning Mrs. Tennessee. Spending a year as Mrs. Tennessee had started to change my life. I was truly beginning to know myself, and I had just started my speaking career. You may wonder why I decided to enter a pageant in my late twenties with a toddler. Sounds ridiculous, right? At the time, I told myself I was just trying to launch a new career.

Looking back, however, I realize that was not the entire truth. I was also looking for personal validation that I was OK. I was looking for a way to feel valued and worthy, because I wasn't wearing my personal crown of self-respect. I still had no real idea of who I was. I was beating myself up for not having a career and being a stay-at-home mom. My low opinion of myself was telling me that I was "just a mom," which I knew was the most important job in the world. I should have viewed it instead like this: I was *chosen* to be Nick Thomas's mom, and this is the greatest job on earth. I was blessed to be home with him during those years. I was blessed to be able to chaperone field trips and be a room mom. I was blessed to take him to school and pick him up. I am proud to say I was and still am a great mom to this special boy who is now an incredible man. But my personal view of myself during those years had me doubting myself and everything that I did. Whether you are a stay-at-home mom or a mom who is working outside the home, the title of *Mom* is the greatest one we will ever have.

I was also in a challenging marriage during those years. We were both very young when we got married, and we didn't understand each other or how to work through very difficult times. I felt very lost and not valued. Instead of working toward building my self-worth from the inside out, I thought winning a pageant would help me feel valued and special. I was looking for outside validation to heal the inner pain of feeling unseen, unheard, and unworthy.

However, it wasn't the crown, the title, or the launch of a career at age thirty that eventually gave me that validation and personal sense of self-worth. It was the internal work I did during that time, and it was the lessons I had to learn along the way—lessons that came through some very hard life experiences, and lessons that were wake-up calls for me to stand up and recognize that I could not wait the rest of my life for external validation. Even if we are fortunate to have outside validation and recognition, it should follow the most important validation of all, and that is the validation from within.

For me, battling low self-esteem and constantly looking for other people to tell me that I was OK eventually took its toll. When you look everywhere else for your value and worth, you stop seeing yourself altogether, and that is exactly what happened to me.

If you do not pay attention to what is going on within, I believe God will get your attention in some way. That day arrived for me when I went in for a yearly routine check-up with my amazing gynecologist and now friend, Dr. Barbara Nylander. As she has done for the twenty-five-plus years I have been her patient, she talked to me about my life and my health. But as we were talking, she was staring at my throat, and she said, "Wait, what is this?" I had no idea what she was talking about. She put her hands to my throat and said in a very shocked voice, "Have you not noticed this? How could you not see this?" She showed me in the mirror this protrusion in my throat that looked like I had swallowed a golf ball. She gave me a very concerned look and said, "Dale, I want you to see a head and neck doctor immediately. This is some type of tumor. I am sure it's nothing to worry about, but you have to find out what is going on."

> 66 *When you look everywhere else for your value and worth, you stop seeing yourself all together.* 99

Looking back, I wonder how it was possible that I could not have seen the growth in my throat. Each day, I was looking in the mirror, brushing my teeth, and doing my makeup and hair, and yet I did not see this big tumor that was protruding from my throat. It seems so symbolic now. I was so lost and unable to see myself that I was unable to see a physical bulge in my throat. It was the second time in my life where I was not aware of what was going on with myself physically because of my internal neglect. I felt invisible and insignificant to others. I was invisible and insignificant in my mind. I now know that there wasn't any way for someone else to see me or understand me when I didn't see myself.

I slowly began to discover what was going on with me physically and it took several years and many different opinions from doctors to come to a conclusion for the best treatment for me. It was a thyroid goiter, which is usually found in much older people and not someone in their thirties. Initially, we thought it could be treated with medication. But because of the size of the goiter, there wasn't a way to biopsy all of it to make sure it wasn't cancer.

After the needle biopsies, ultrasounds, and finally finding the right doctor, the decision was made to go in and remove the entire thyroid gland with the tumor. I was reminded they couldn't be sure it wasn't cancer. I was also reminded over and over again that it was near my vocal chords and there could be a risk of my vocal chords being damaged. I remember being so scared as I was lying there alone, about to be rolled into surgery. I had just started my speaking career; I had just started to "find" my voice, both internally and externally, and I was being told there was a small chance that during surgery that could be taken away. But my faith was stronger than my fear. I truly believed God had given me the dream of being a speaker and He would see me through this surgery. I had to adopt the same belief with my health as I do the weather forecast. It may be 20 percent chance of rain, but that is 80 percent chance of sun.

During the journey to seek out the right physicians for my physical health issue, I knew it was time I got serious about looking at what was going on with my inner soul that had caused me not to be able to see the tumor that was so obvious to everyone else. I found an incredible therapist to guide me through that continued personal discovery to find Dale—the Dale who had truly gotten lost along the way. I had started the journey to personal growth in my mid-twenties but had not stayed consistent with it after becoming a new mom. I had to understand the Dale who felt invisible and very unsafe. I had to get 100 percent committed to the inner work that I continue to do even today. I took the time and read the books, sought out expert teachers, and began to ask myself the tough questions.

I realized it was not a coincidence that my body had been attacked where I felt the weakest. I began to understand the true connection between my emotional well-being and the well-being of my body. I began to understand the messages I had continued to tell myself over and over again. I had believed that I couldn't speak up for myself and that my opinions were not valid, and that it was my throat where I faced the health challenge. It was Louise Hay's book *You Can Heal Your Life* that spoke to me in such a strong way during this journey and began to show me those emotional connections to what was going on in my physical body.

Although it took years, I emerged from that experience both physically and emotionally healthier and stronger. I chose to not only face my diagnosis and challenges but to learn from them. I began to trust myself and my inner voice. The tumor was not cancer, but a scan showed other small tumors on my right thyroid gland. I was told that I would need to be on thyroid medication for the rest of my life to control it.

After a short time on the medication, I was experiencing side effects and not feeling well. I felt deep in my soul that the medication wasn't right for me. I shared how I was feeling with a friend who happens to be a doctor, and he suggested that I totally come off the medication to see how my body would react. He thought my body might simply adjust. My body seemed to know exactly what to do, and my right thyroid gland began functioning as if I had both glands. It's been seventeen years, and my single thyroid gland is still doing the work for two. I am continually amazed at the power of the body to heal.

Those years were some of the most transformational years of my life. They were not easy years, but growth is usually never easy. I had to take a very honest look at myself and everything I believed. I had to learn to trust myself and my instinct. I had to face the fear and uncertainty I felt, and I had to trust the faith that my life has been built on. I had to take a strong look at my life and decide to take control of my physical and emotional well-being. It was a scary time in my life, but I allowed it to refine me, make me stronger, and let it help me learn more about myself.

> **66***I survived because the fire inside me burned brighter than the fire around me.***99**

JOSHUA GRAHAM

After those few years of uncertainty, I came out physically healthy and whole, but my marriage did not survive. Going through that scary and uncertain experience, I needed support and encouragement that my husband could not provide. As I began to dig deeper personally, I realized that we were not healthy for each other and had not been for a long time. Ending my fifteen-year marriage to the father of my son was one of the hardest decisions I have ever made. I am proud to say that even though our relationship as husband and wife didn't continue, we have found a new respect for each other through the years and have emerged as friends and great parents to Nick.

In the last chapter, we talked about darkness and light. During that time, darkness and doubt told me that I would get sick and not survive. Faith and light told me that there wasn't a diagnosis yet—it was a "potential" diagnosis. Doubt told me that I wasn't valuable and being single at forty would be miserable. Faith told me it wasn't true, my relationship status had nothing to do with my value, and each day was a new beginning to be all I was called to be.

In my experience, it seems that women struggle a great deal with their self-worth when it comes to dealing with men. I have heard women over and over again ask this question: "Why is he treating me this way?" As Dr. Phil says, "Why do they treat you that way? Because they can." Think about that answer. "Because they can." What does that mean? It means if we feel we are not being treated fairly, it is up to us to set the boundary for ourselves.

How many times through the years as women have we tried every way in the world to prove to a man that we were the "right one" or that we were "special enough" for him to look our way? How many times have we asked these questions: "What is wrong with me? Why doesn't he like me? Why doesn't he text me back like he said he would? Why isn't he calling me back? Why is he treating me this way?" I know I have done it.

Remember, *no* man can ever give you your self-worth, but you can allow any man to rob you of it. Each time a man doesn't return your call or respond to you and you ask yourself "What is wrong with me?" you are asking the wrong question. Of course, we always need to evaluate and make sure we are taking responsibility for our part in the relationship. We can all improve ourselves daily, and I believe we should. But those questions are *all* the wrong questions. They are questions that are questioning our value and our worth. I think the questions should be more of a personal exploration: "Why are you allowing it to happen to you? Is he valuable enough to you? Do you want someone in your life who can't keep his word even to return a phone call? Do you want someone in your life to whom you have to beg for the attention and emotional support you deserve?

If someone shows you who they are through their words and actions, believe them the first time! Stop trying to rewrite the story into something it's not. Stop making excuses for bad behavior. When you excuse bad behavior, you then accept the consequences that come with that decision. Your question should always be, "Does this make me feel more or less valuable?" If it makes you feel less valuable, take a hard look and ask yourself why you are making those actions acceptable. Make sure your crown hasn't fallen on the floor! If you want to make a change in your life, you have to take 100 percent responsibility for yourself and what you accept in your life.

You have to ask yourself the tough questions. What has happened that has caused me to feel this way? What was said to me or what action was taken that caused me to feel this way? What am I choosing to think, feel, and accept that has taken my personal value away today? It takes a strong (not hard, but strong), secure, valuable woman to walk away from being treated less than she deserves. You must evaluate all of your relationships: friends, work, family, and love. Especially in love relationships, I see women stay in a place where they are not valued because they have convinced themselves that their partner is someone they can't live without.

When you start to feel invisible, defeated, unattractive, and like you are not valuable, *halt*. One of the greatest lessons I have ever learned is the word *HALT*. If you are *Hungry, Angry, Lonely,* or *Tired*, then you need to give yourself a time-out. Do not make big decisions, do not take action—HALT! Stop and tune in. Take a deep breath. Listen to your soul. Listen to what you are saying to yourself. Are you taking someone's actions or his or her opinion of you and making it your reality? If you are, then HALT. There is one thing you can change in that situation; you can change your mind. You can find the invisible crown that you have misplaced.

> **"** *If you want to make a change in your life,*
> *you have to take 100 percent responsibility for*
> *yourself and what you accept in your life.* **"**

How do you change what I like to refer to as the lost crown syndrome? When we lose sight of who we are, we lose sight of our boundaries, and we start to accept "good enough" as "enough." You have to stand up and see yourself as the valuable woman you are. We are first-rate women, and we have to stop trying to convince ourselves that being treated less than that is not a crime against our souls. When we surrender our self-respect over and over again, it begins to feel normal, and we expect it—it becomes a self-fulfilling prophecy.

> **"** *It takes a strong (not hard, but strong),*
> *secure, valuable woman to walk away from*
> *being treated less than she deserves.* **"**

If you want to be loved, adored, supported, encouraged, seen, heard, admired, respected, and treasured, then you have to step up and hold out for those who will treat you that way. If you are giving away time, space, and energy to those who are not treating you with value and respect, then they are taking up space for someone who could treat you that way. If you are spending all of your time trying to get someone to pay attention to you, then you are missing the ones who will. Let it go. Release it. Clear space. A true queen who is generous in heart and spirit would never allow herself to be treated that way, so why would you?

When you truly begin to love and respect the woman that God created you to be, then you will not allow anyone to disrespect her. Treat yourself as you would your daughter. You would not stand by and allow your daughter to be disrespected or her self-worth challenged, so do not do it to yourself. In the midst of confusion and chaos, pause and be still. In the middle of fear and doubt, be still, know, and remember who you are. Replace your doubt, fear, and uncertainty with knowledge and confidence. You can't desire something in your life and expect to receive it when you only focus on the absence of it.

It seems that many times when we are not feeling seen or heard, we keep pushing, trying to find a way for someone to validate us. I read a comment recently by the actress Julianne Moore that spoke volumes to me. She said, "People feel the least present when they don't feel seen. It's impossible to be present when no one sees you. And it becomes a self-perpetuating process, because the more that people don't acknowledge you, the more you feel you don't exist. There's no space for you. Conversely, you are the most present when you are the most seen."

Just in the past few years, I have started to recognize and understand that one of the deepest desires of my soul is to be "seen" and "heard." What does that mean? It means that someone takes the time and interest to not just listen to you when you speak but to truly hear you. There are many people who listen but never hear.

There are many people who look but never see. There are many people who touch but never feel.

When someone takes the time and has the desire to truly "know you" at an authentic level—to know your heart, your soul, and your fears—you have been seen. When someone truly sees you and knows you at a deeper level, there is no judgment; there is only acceptance. It's not about who you are or what you do or what you can do for that person. It's simply about being. You can't make someone see you, and you can't make someone hear you. Either they do, or they don't. The feeling of really being seen and understood gives you the power to stand in your personal presence and expand even more.

Whether anyone else sees you or hears you is not within your control. But what is within your control is that *you* see yourself and hear yourself. Those desires that are deep in your heart need you to hear them. They need your attention. They need you to acknowledge them. Don't walk away from what you want and what you know you need in your life just because some other person does not recognize it. Stand up for you. Be strong for you. Give those deep desires of your heart the same love and respect you want from others.

I truly believe that once you start to honor yourself and you are no longer focused on what is lacking in your life, then amazingly the support you need will also appear in the form of a friend, a teacher, a partner, or someone in your life. When you stop knocking on closed doors, you will begin to see windows and doors that are open and waiting for you to recognize them. When you focus on the people that you feel are not showing up for you, then you are giving them that attention and the space that could be occupied by those who would support you. It's not fair to them, and it's not fair to you. They can't give you what they don't have.

One of my favorite books, *Zero Point Agreement,* was recommended to me by my best friend. One of the most powerful things

I read in this book was, "Stop going to the hardware store for fruit salad." Wow! Let that sink in. Stop going to people who can't or choose not to meet your needs to get your needs met. It's like going to the hardware store for fruit salad. Love and accept people for who they are and what they bring to your life. Let go of the expectations and expect more of yourself than anyone else.

Stop focusing on the people who don't see you and start looking for the ones who do. They are out there, and once you find those who will be that believing mirror in your life, your life will begin to change in a way you can't imagine. Learn to see yourself as the valuable person you are, and surround yourself with people who will lift you higher.

Even though I teach and share these messages, there are still days I feel depleted and need that reminder. We need someone who can truly see past our exterior and see the truth in our souls. I still need people in my life who lift me higher and encourage me to keep my crown on my head. I am so blessed to have a small tribe of true friends who truly know me and see me. They lovingly remind me when I am too tired, too emotionally exhausted, and too depleted to be my personal best. They remind me of who I am and point it out to me when life has taken its toll and I start to take the first sip of doubt—when my crown is sliding. We will all continue to face times of doubt. It's not about not facing those times; it's about how long will we allow ourselves to stay in that place.

> ❝ *Stop focusing on the people who don't see you.* ❞

Have you ever doubted your self-worth? What about your value? Have you doubted your ability? Get tough with yourself and discover what you have allowed that has caused you to step into the belief that you are not worthy. Your soul is mourning the fact that you have walked away from the queen that you are. Your soul is mourning the fact that you have allowed your crown to fall off too many times. If you have allowed someone to steal your self-worth (and we all have), then forgive yourself and forgive them. It's not the statement of "forgive and forget." You can forget exactly what was done to you, but do *not* forget the lessons that were learned through that experience.

Queens are never victims—they are victors. They turn pain into the power of learning. They know that at every moment they still have a choice in how they respond. They are not defeated—they are defined and refined by each experience that didn't bring the result they wanted or that caused them pain. Queens are soul-directed and purpose-driven.

I want to remind you once again, *yes,* you are a queen. The dictionary says a queen is a woman of supreme rank, power, or attractiveness who rules a kingdom in her right. You do own a kingdom of your right; it is the kingdom of *you.* Think about it right now: you are a gorgeous queen with a divine purpose to be all you were created to be. You are unique, talented, strong, and gorgeous, and you are *enough*!

> 66 *To all the girls who no longer believe in fairy tales and happy endings: You are the writer of this story. Chin up and straighten your crown; you are the queen of this kingdom, and only you know how to rule it.* 99

B. DEVINE

You have talents that only you have. You have a purpose on this planet that only you have. If you do not fulfill your destiny and your purpose, then no one else can fulfill it. The book that you feel you are supposed to write can only be *your* book. That song you are supposed to sing is only *your* song. That business you feel led to start is only *your* business. If you do not make the decision to follow that dream, that prompting in your soul, then that dream and that work will leave this planet with you. It's *only* yours.

We have to remind each other in our sisterhood that we should always hold our well-being sacred. Real beauty, the kind of beauty that is not affected by age or anything else on this earth, is the beauty that comes from your mind, not from your mirror.

One of my favorite passages seems to be the perfect way to bring *Good Morning Gorgeous* to a close. Thank you, F. Scott Fitzgerald, for these perfect words. This is for all of you. I hope you will read these words and reread them until they become a part of your mind, heart, and soul.

> 66 *She was beautiful, but not like those girls in the magazines. She was beautiful, for the way she thought. She was beautiful, for that sparkle in her eyes when she talked about something she loved. She was beautiful, for her ability to make other people smile even if she was sad. No, she wasn't beautiful for something as temporary as her looks. She was beautiful, deep down to her soul.* 99

F. SCOTT FITZGERALD

Here we are at the last moment of this book together. I am so grateful you took the time to be here, to learn, to explore, and to expand your mind. I told you in the beginning I wanted to give you a gift for taking this journey with me. Simply email me at Dale@winnersbychoice.com and mention the GMG free gift, and I will send it to you.

In this book, I have shared with you the ideas that have changed my life, and now you have the opportunity to change your life. It only takes one idea to truly steer your life in a different direction, but you have to put that idea into action. You make changes in every area of your life by changing *you*! The good news and bad news is it truly is up to you and only you! No one can make the changes in your life but you. You are one real decision away from creating the life you want, the life you deserve, the life that is filled with peace and happiness. Are you ready to make that decision starting right here and right now? I believe that you are!

So, to all of you, my Good Morning Gorgeous Sisterhood, I say, "Crown up! The world needs you and is waiting for you. Take your gifts and share them, and encourage others to find and pursue their gifts. Join with me, and let's all be ambassadors of light and love. Welcome to the Good Morning Gorgeous Tribe; together we can change the world one gorgeous soul at a time!"

66 *Beauty begins the moment you decide to be yourself.* 99

COCO CHANEL

66 *We ask ourselves, 'Who am I to be brilliant, gorgeous, talented, fabulous?' Actually, who are you not to be?* 99

MARIANNE WILLIAMSON

Take Aways

_____

_____

_____

_____

_____

_____

_____

_____

_____

_____

_____

_____

_____

_____

_____

_____

Acknowledgments

As I come to the end of this journey of writing this book, I just have to thank God for the incredible opportunities I have had to share my message around the world over the past twenty-plus years. I could truly never have imagined the life I now live. It brings me to tears each time I hear from someone in my audience that my message has made a difference. I know that I am just the messenger, and I am just so thankful to have been given this gift. I will honor it and will never take it for granted.

For everyone who has inspired me, challenged me, encouraged me, and pushed me in the creation of this book, you will never truly understand how much I appreciate you. It is with a grateful heart to my followers, my readers, my team, and my family and friends that I offer you my heartfelt thanks. You will never know how you have changed my life.

About the Author

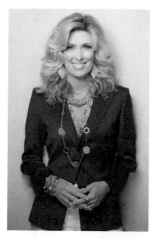

Dale Smith Thomas is the president and founder of Winners By Choice, Inc. and an international motivational speaker and author. Dale's empowering, enlightening, and entertaining message has challenged and inspired hundreds of thousands of people around the world to choose success in all areas of their lives.

In addition to traveling the world as an empowerment speaker, Dale is a frequent guest on radio and television. She has been a featured guest on *The Dr. Phil Show, The Big Idea* on CNBC, the Travel Channel, CMT, MTV, and VH1. She was also featured on a reality show on the Fox network.

Dale is a self-described unapologetic optimist, and her passion for making a difference is stamped on every page of her life. Pulling from her real-life experiences growing up in North Mississippi, Dale shares real life lessons that give you the tools to be your personal best.

Her client list reads like a Who's Who, but her lasting impact is with her audience members. Her "I've known you all my life" personality has her audience members walking away with a new belief that they can truly achieve their dreams. As one of her audience members stated, "Your name should read Dale Smith Thomas, PHD, The Hope Doctor."

Dale is a Mississippi native who now makes her home in Nashville, TN.

Be sure to sign up for Dale's weekly newsletter, her podcast, and her YouTube presentations. Follow her on social media. For all links and information about booking Dale for speaking engagements and appearances, visit www.WinnersByChoice.com

Take Aways

_____

_____

_____

_____

_____

_____

_____

_____

_____

_____

_____

_____

_____

_____

_____

_____

_____

_____

Take Aways

_____

_____

_____

_____

_____

_____

_____

_____

_____

_____

_____

_____

_____

_____

_____

_____

Take Aways

_____

_____

_____

_____

_____

_____

_____

_____

_____

_____

_____

_____

_____

_____

_____

_____